Surviving Polarity
In Poems and Pictures

Joe Smith

WALDENHOUSE PUBLISHERS, INC.
WALDEN, TENNESSEE

Surviving Polarity in Poems and Pictures

Type and design by Karen Paul Stone
Published by Waldenhouse Publishers, Inc.
100 Clegg Street, Signal Mountain, Tennessee 37377 USA
423-886-2721 www.waldenhouse.com
Printed in the United States of America
ISBN: 978-1-947589-77-3
Library of Congress Control Number: 2024930908

An anthology of poems written from the viewpoint of a bipolar poet covering topics such as Bipolar symptoms, personal preference humor, disappointment, poetic efforts including types and techniques, tributes to a few professionals, dreams, and miscellaneous topics. - Provided by publisher

POE023000 POETRY / Subjects & Themes / General
HEA055000 HEALTH & FITNESS / Mental Health
SEL020010 SELF-HELP / Mood Disorders / Bipolar Disorder

To

This, my second book of collected poems,
is dedicated to my remaining brothers and sisters
who have done so much for me over the years.

Ruth Helen Rudolph
Victor Ulysses Smith
Dennis Jameson Smith
Kirby Louis Bernard Smith
Frances Lebre Decker
Patricia Marie Darnell
Alice Maureen Cobbs
Ferol Teresa Whitworth

Endorsements

Based on Life Between The Poles

Joseph Smith is an excellent wordsmith. He has the unique ability to intrigue his readers and push the reader along to the next line. Joe's thoughtful penmanship delves into his own psyche, while passively urging the reader to begin his own journey.

- Bob Hopkins

Joe's poetry paints vibrant pictures bringing the reader intense feelings.

- Martha Rankin

You can't run and you can't hide for awhile, so release your feelings and get on with Life.

-Ronald G. Smith

I was blessed to read poems presented from Joe Smith's book, *Life Between The Poles.* His poetry leads me down paths of memory and imagination.

- Joyce Fox

Contents

CHAPTER ONE
Exploring Polarity

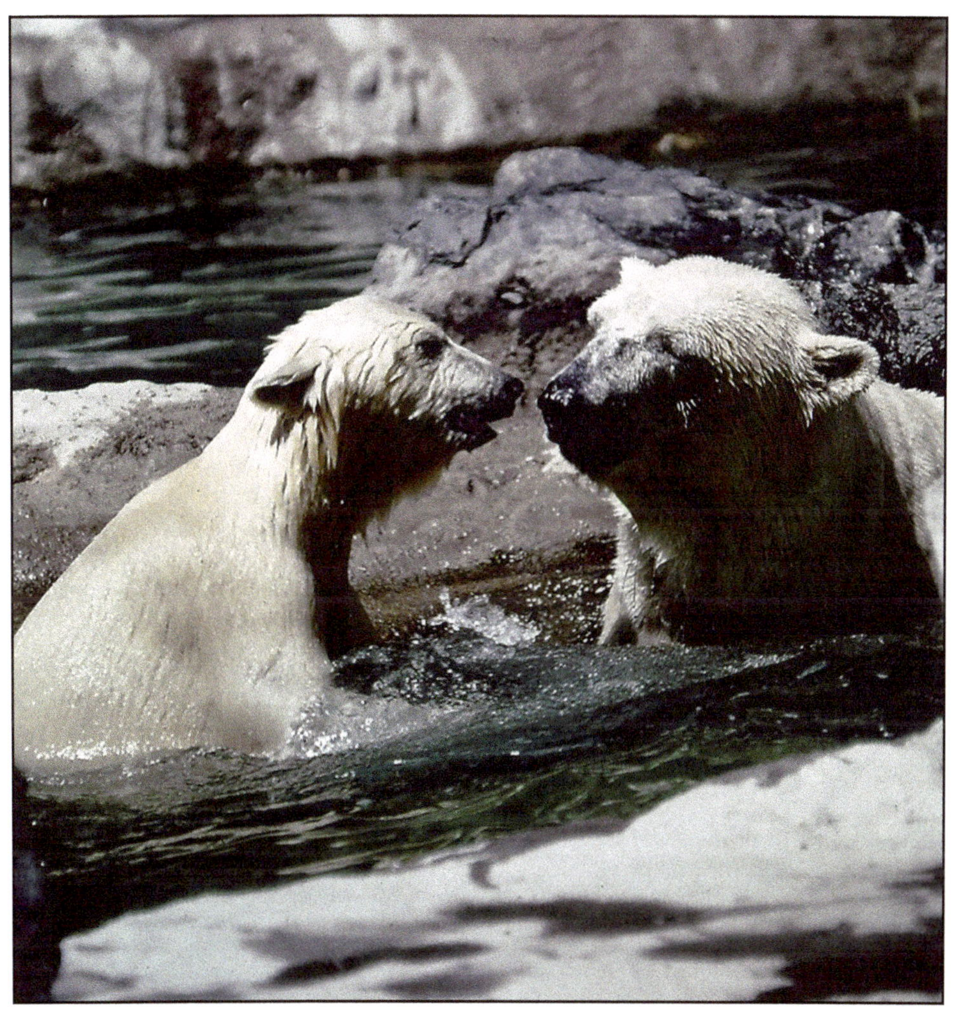

Traveling on the Polar Express

When the train first leaves the station
There's no need for preoccupation
All needed faculties are on board
Anti-psychotics, no need to hoard

But somewhere along the way
The mind games start to play
Here we make allusion
To the onset of delusion

Objects outside the train
May slowly fade and wane
The scenery loses its appeal
And the impossible seems real

It seems possible to multitask
But effectiveness, it seems, won't last
Thoughts, it seems, come ever faster
But the simple things I cannot master

When the train is going fast
People appear, some from the past
Some I've never seen before
Others bring me frights galore

And when the train gains more speed
The doctor's word I fail to heed
I simply shun the Pullman Car
No sleep I need though I travel far

The caravan begins to pick up speed
And inside it becomes hard to read
Concentration starts to fail
And the train runs off the rails

A crane is called to right the train
The organized correction causes pain
The patient sings a sad refrain
Because he knows he's not quite sane

Once the train's back on the track
I declare I won't come back
But then another issue arises
Riding this train is full of surprises

The locomotive then enters a long dark tunnel
Into my mind thoughts start to funnel
Deep regrets and events from the past
It seems that things don't move so fast

My mind slows down, and starts to dwell
On all the things I've not done well
I feel blue and kind of empty
These feelings start at the tunnel entry

Other issues come to mind
If I'd ignore them I'd be blind
Friends and kin who've left the train
Generate some of the pain

My thoughts turn toward the Terminal
If I go there all might be well
But the price of admittance could be my soul
Not a very good deal on the whole

And so again I call for the crew
This gets old, there's nothing new
I'm trundled off to the station
Where pills and doctors are awaitin'

So I travel down the track
And know full well that I'll be back

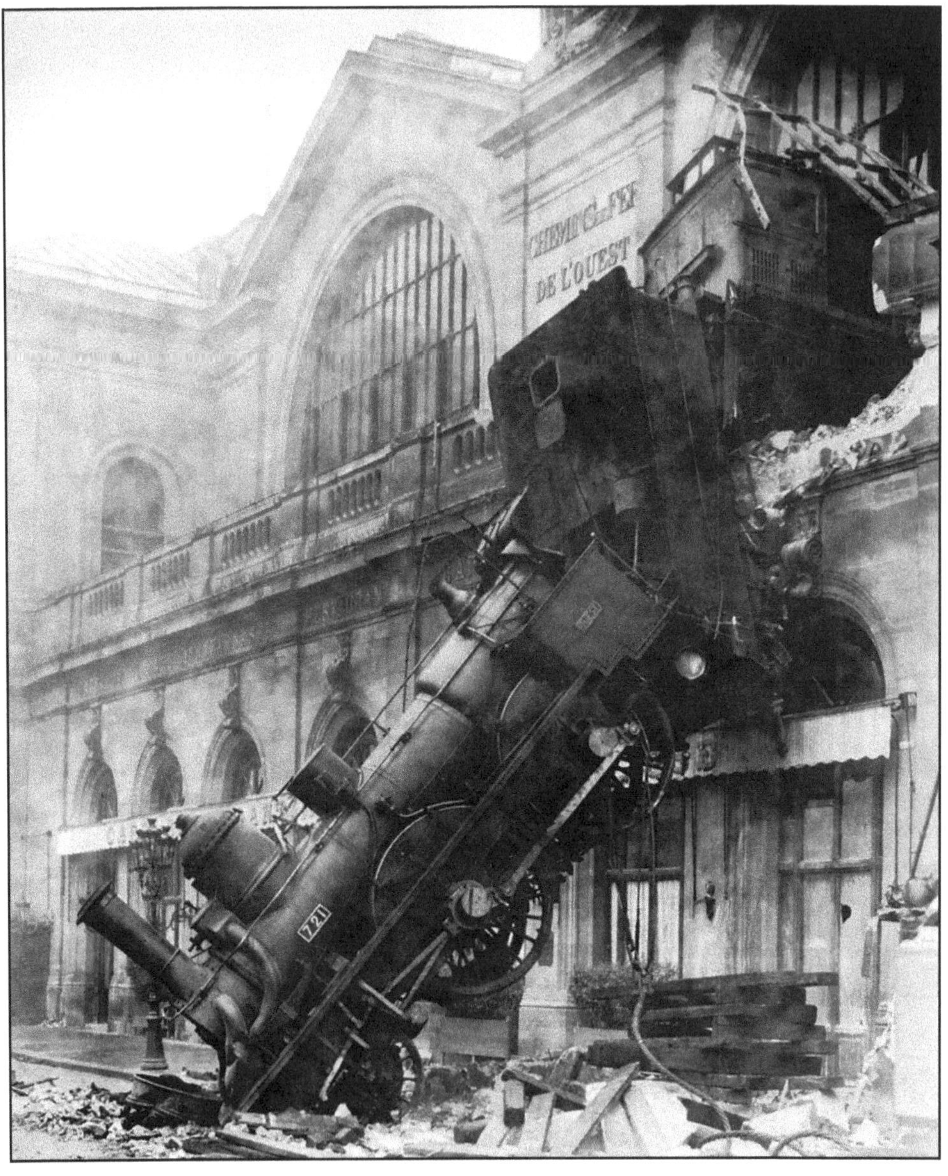

The Polar Express Under Duress

Joe Smith

Beware The Big Bad Wolf

Many are the times I log
Fighting off the big black dog
The time it seems to me is wasted
So seldom is a victory tasted

No matter what I try to do
Can't erase the mood so blue
In addition to the joy I lack
Is the fear that he'll come back

Yes, chasing off a down turned mood
Is a chore I have very often pursued
Scaring off the big black dog
By managing the mental fog

But often times the dog, that baleful beast
Is relieved by an ancestor that wants me deceased
My chances of survival are severely decreased
As the controlling thoughts of the wolf are released

Yes there are times when the black dog is joined
By the wolf by whom my will to live is purloined
He hunts his prey in fields of thoughts most uncertain
Hopes to be the agent of doom who rings down my curtain

There are situations of which he takes advantage
Realms of reason perverted in which he does damage
He often loves to feed off of unfounded guilt
Through which he causes my life force to wilt

He also has a taste for the unintended slight
Which he pounces on with all of his might
Though hurt or insult were never my intention
Attempts to self forgive are never in contention

Particularly tasty to him is the odd mistake
The embarrassment of which I can't shake
Because I did a thing incorrectly
I'm punished for it quite directly

Sometimes simply my overall situation
My stature in life, my social station
These can lead to dissatisfaction
Which tempt the wolf in another fashion

The wolf takes me in his jaws
And my life seems a lost cause
I twist and turn to make my escape
My salvation thereby I try to shape

I employ my silver bullets it's true
And that's not the only thing I do
To keep the dog and wolf at bay
To try and last another day

I remind myself that death and then eternity
Spent without means of escape from the wolf would be
Far worse than managing life with uncertainty
Brought on by the wolf and the wish not to be

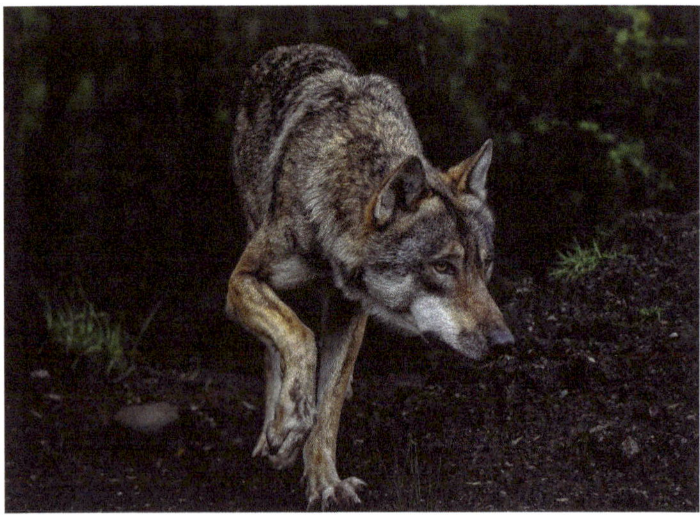

The Big Bad Wolf

Joe Smith

Definitely Delusional

I've chosen here to make an allusion
To a mistaken notion we call a delusion
Despite evidence in support of the contrary
The mind can make acceptance necessary

Yes the mind simply performs an illusion
And presents as fact the current delusion
You see, everything about it seems real
Controls how you think and how you feel

Delusion coupled with acute paranoia
Can cripple you quick, really annoy ya'
Try as you might you just can't believe
Facts as presented; the delusions deceive

As a result of the messy mental malfunction
You're presented with a clear compunction
You can't help yourself you have to believe
The delusion's tenets, there is no reprieve

The acceptance of the delusions leads to further action
This in response to the fully formed deluded faction
You give away your wealth, you think there's no future
You suffer war wounds that no surgeon can suture

All this flies in the face of advice from your friends
Despite your best efforts the threat never ends
You try to believe what your friends try to tell you
In the back of your mind you doubt what they'd sell you

The delusion comes and may last for days
It's often evil and wicked in its ways
It occupies the mind, pushes out other thoughts
It grips the psyche and ties it up in knots

It's sometimes scary and even pernicious
Unkind in all respects and even vicious
It's complete in its preoccupation
Uncertain as it is in its duration

Sometimes the delusion can take on a positive bent
Though I've never known one to which this facet is lent
I'm used to all my delusions with scary intent
In an atmosphere of dread they're left to ferment

But in the end the delusion frequently is cleared
Often with none of the consequences feared
But in each case there's a price to be paid
If nothing else, that peace of mind is delayed

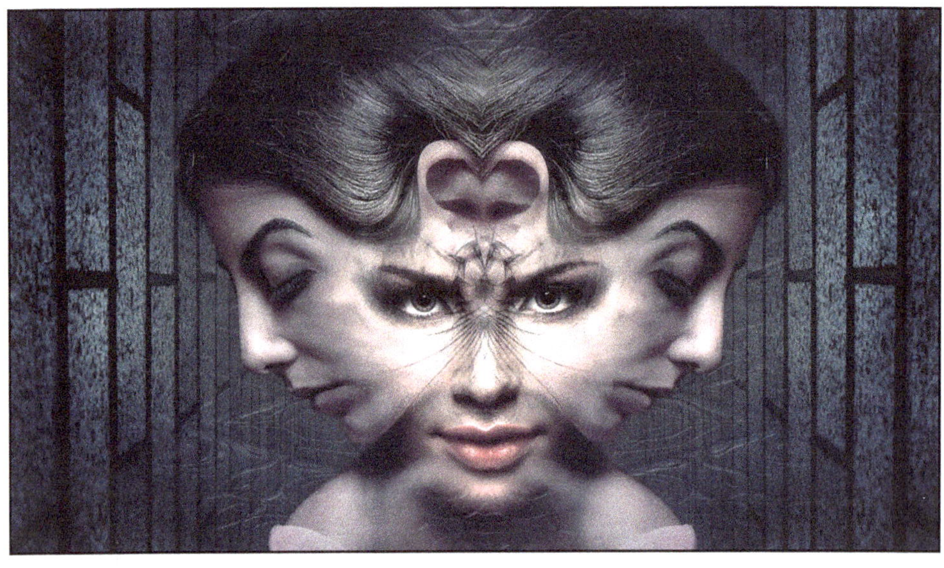

Laboring Under a Delusion

Joe Smith

Hallucinations

It seems like imagination
Under control of automation
Without clear indication
Bends the rules of observation

It's an unusual situation
Requires no concentration
Yes, automatic generation
Doesn't pass investigation

It's always perceived in isolation
Yet sometimes yields conversation
May include a wild sensation
Often ends in deep frustration

May be tied to occupation
Often wrapped in insulation
Sometimes full of exaggeration
Always subject to interpretation

From reality there's separation
But there may be some correlation
What's required is mere translation
Something less than inculcation

Requires a bit of discrimination
May affect one's reputation
Defining calls for cooperation
Equal views, no subjugation

It's a case of aberrant visualization
Sometimes results in hospitalization
Calls for careful communication
Comes from psychic fragmentation

Indicative of mental decentralization
Part and parcel of psycho animation
Seeking now no dispensation
Knowing here no affirmation

Resulting at times in humiliation
Always found with fascination
With discovery comes emancipation
And then comes sensory cessation

Sometimes causes palpitation
Depending on the association
Episodes require evaluation
Often tend toward sensation

Usually denies refutation
Despite obvious aberration
Relation leads to augmentation
Results in considerable consternation

Prescription leads to mitigation
Reduces phantom creation
Helps provide illumination
In a given application

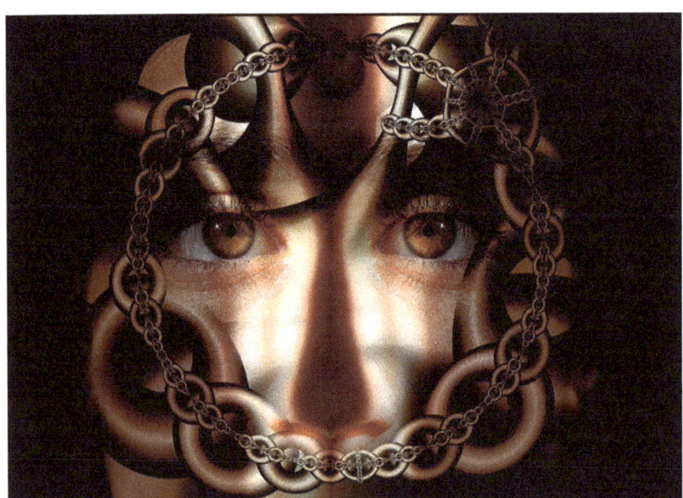

A Hellish Hallucination

Insomnia II

When I went to bed last night
I wasn't feeling just quite right
I really wasn't feeling sleepy
What I felt was kind of creepy

And as I lay me down to sleep
Into my mind thoughts would creep
It did no good to try and stop them
My efforts failed to try and drop them

It wasn't that my conscience bothered
And no childish thoughts were fathered
It simply seemed a general unease
That my disquieted mind would seize

A feeling that I was trapped
And all my initiative was sapped
Stuck between a rock and hard place
I tried to struggle out of this space

No matter which way I turned
My try at extrication was spurned
As my efforts at resolution increased
My energy was at last deceased

I found myself just dwelling
On a subject quite compelling
Of two options I could choose
With either one I would lose

It seems no matter which path I choose
There's one I'll hurt and one I'll bruise
I never meant to cause anyone pain
As I sought sleep I heard this refrain

This all started when I was manic
And it turned into a virtual panic
I sure can't say I saw it coming
Didn't seem wrong to be forthcoming

But by letting my feelings show
I let the animus and discord grow
It certainly wasn't my intention
To sew the seeds of dissension

And so now I find myself here
What I should do next isn't clear
From my dreams there came no clues
It looks as if I must pay my dues

So tonight I'll try again
A new trend to begin
And if again I don't sleep
Into the depths I will creep

I'm stuck, it seems, there is no doubt
I just can't seem to work this out
There's just no way I can explain
Without causing them more pain

I wish this situation would go away
But it's here, it seems, to stay
It doesn't matter how I feel
With it, it seems, I must deal

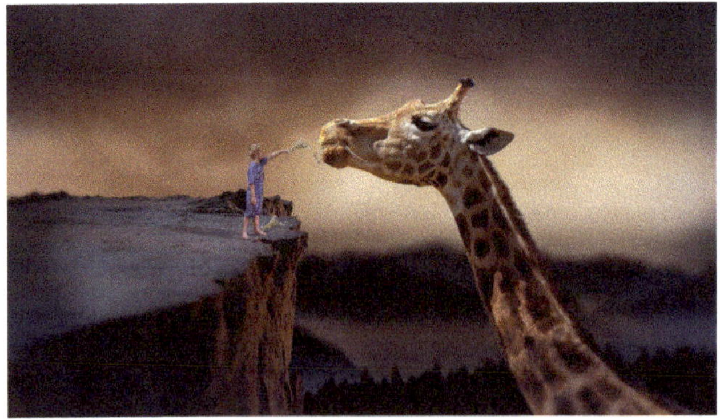

If An Insomniac Could Dream

Night Time Delusions

I had a dream the other night
A tapestry of illusions
Something about it wasn't right
A patchwork of delusions

I didn't understand it quite
The cast was unfamiliar
As I said, it wasn't right
Neither saga nor a thriller

It simply was a case
Of worrisome conflict
People rushing to and fro
No attempts to interdict

I recognized my old workplace
It hadn't changed that much
I found myself in my old space
With desk and tools and such

But the manager was not my last one
But rather one from long ago
I didn't understand why a past one
Was pacing to and fro

Pacing was typically an indicator
That all was not quite right
He behaved just like a dictator
At least he did that night

Strangers occupied
The remainder of my dream
The cause of the consternation
Wasn't in my conscious stream

So I found myself confronting
An unknown mysterious puzzle
Solution to this mystery I was hunting
While wearing a barbed wire muzzle

No facts had been presented
As to what the problem was
And I had not consented
To remediate the cause

But responsibility was assigned
To me and me alone
To a problem undefined
All I could do was groan

As the dream progressed
And hurtled towards conclusion
The point of it digressed
And drowned in the delusions

A problem it seemed existed
But could not be defined
Resolution was thus resisted
No solution was refined

While I contemplated my position
The dream came to an end
Some form of job sedition
No notes to append

And so it was that I awoke
Not solving the problem at hand
My best skill sets I did evoke
The solution was not at my command

So in the end I had no solution
To the problem that was not defined
I simply made no contribution
To abject failure I was resigned

But even though the task was impossible
Since the problem was nowhere described
Somehow I still felt responsible
For a solution that wasn't fully prescribed

And so I was left with a feeling
Of weakness and impotence
By a semi-conscious series of being
A creature of incompetence

So the experience left me reeling
With a feeling of low self esteem
I couldn't rid myself of this feeling
Even though it was just a dream

There's not much to this story
From beginning to the end
There's certainly no glory
Of that I won't pretend

Medication brings on the dreams
But guarantees no good one
Conflict then is all, it seems
Resolution thus it will shun

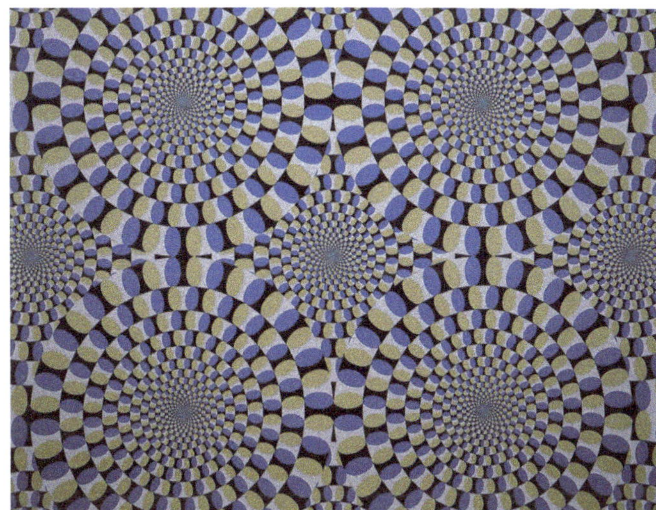

A Delusion of Irritation

Night Time Delusions Followup

I've been assigned an exercise
To complete it I must fantasize
To add facts where none exist
In fantasy I must persist

To create a problem to solve
And this problem to resolve
So problem defined and then solution
While avoiding dreaded word pollution

The problem needs to be about work
A place where many tend to lurk
I'm having trouble defining one
But I'll develop one before I'm done

Most of the problems I had were technical
Which don't lend themselves to this spectacle
So I'll have to conceive of something simple
An example that will provide a symbol

Let's say that the issue involves recording
Series of numbers that come from measuring
The problem being frequent transposition
Entering digits in the wrong position

This problem is a common one
Solving it will mean we're done
Transcription errors in dimensions
Solution must cause no apprehensions

That is to say it must be simple to use
Easily implemented with steps not too obtuse
A system that requires little to no planning
On the technician's part, maybe auto scanning?

So I started a project to review software
And found an option that existed there
What it was was a Generic Gauge Interface
That was automatic; manual entry it would replace

All our gauges had internal data ports
Connecting to computers to make reports
Transposition would be a thing of the past
And the system would be lightning fast

The new gauging system was implemented
Corporate QA reviewed it and complimented
The system and the implementation
It was rolled out through the organization

Turns out I didn't have to fabricate
This story of mine to relate
You see the story is true
Not made up out of the blue

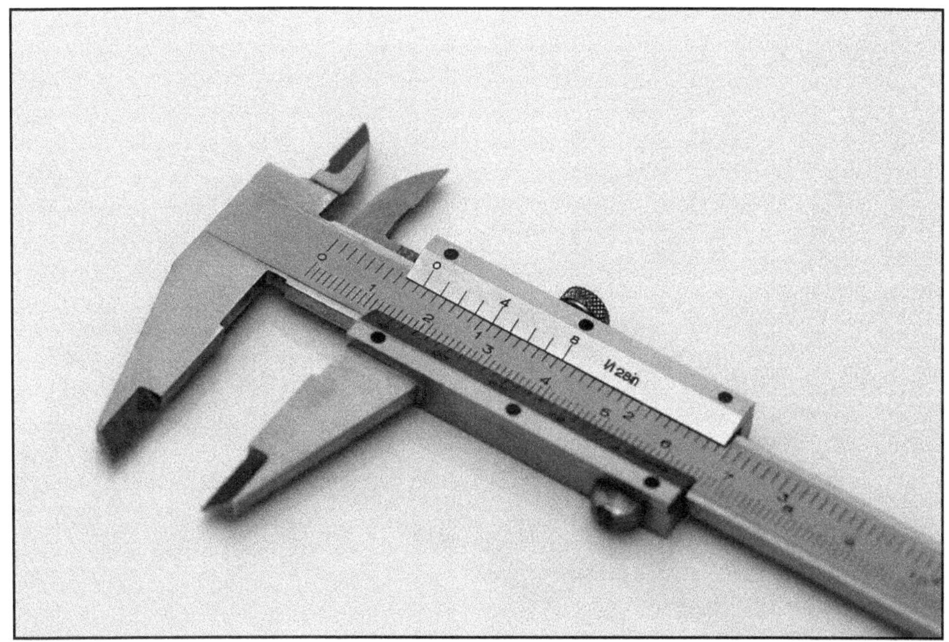

Measuring Up

CHAPTER TWO
Dislikes

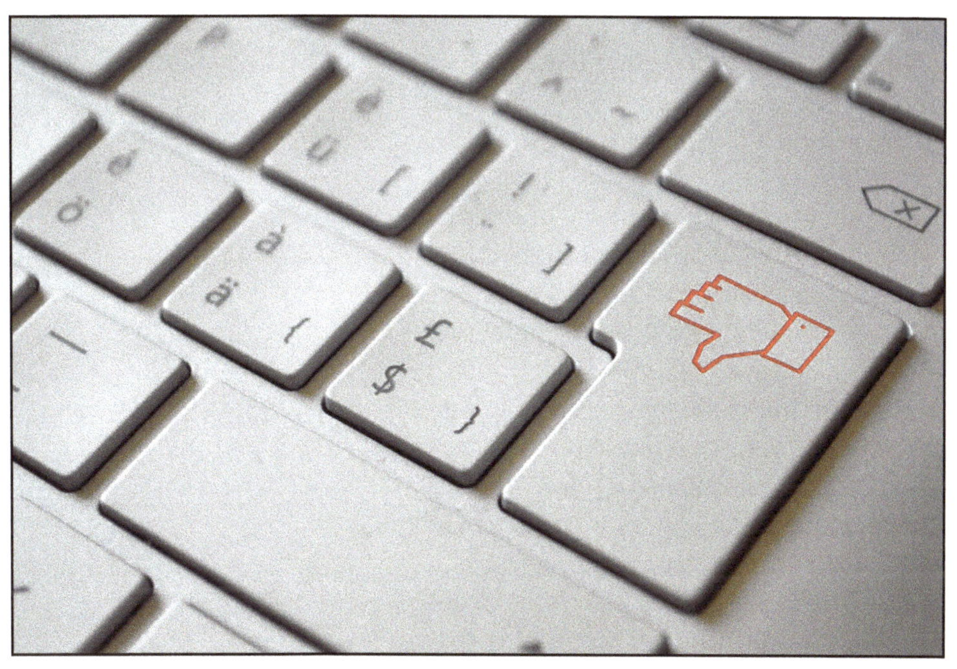

Identifying Your Dislikes Is Key

Ballad of the Big Bad Banana

I've done my best to make it known
That there is not a banana grown
That can even begin to tease me
Much less ever hope to please me

Bananas, you know, I have always said
Were invented just to fill me with dread
Their main purpose, you see, is to gag maggots
The original cause of upturned noses in rabbits

My first objection is to the gross texture
Often disguised by a peanut butter mixture
Next in line of objection is the sickening aroma
Effect of which is to induce a life threatening coma

And then we come to the issue of ripening
Which, in itself, is somewhat frightening
The banana starts out hard and green
Then turns black with yellow seldom seen

Yellow, I'm told, is banana's true gold
The condition in which it's hope they're sold
But nothing, it seems, controls the palette
Variation alone causes failure on the first ballot

After consumption there's the issue of banana detritus*
Of course a concern only second to possible gastritis
Once consumed there's the matter of old peel disposal
Preventing slippage on the offal is a whole new proposal

What other fruit, I ask, has such a reputation
For causing accidents due to disposal violation
And what fruit degraded is in bread compiled
Nay, I say, no other fresh fruit is so reviled

* waste or debris

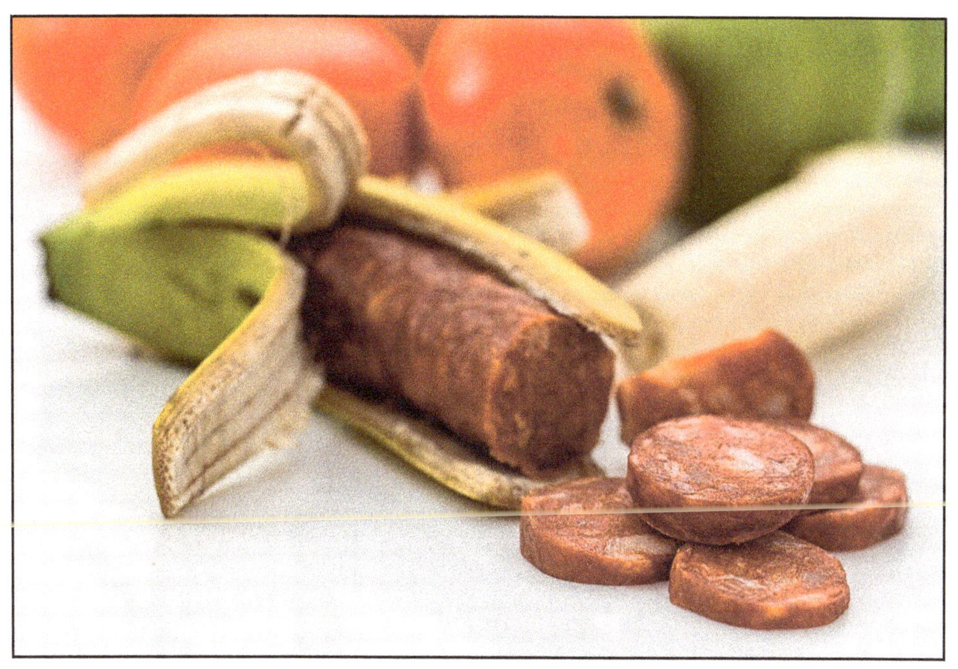

A Banana I Can Appreciate

The Odyssey

This is the tale of an onerous oddity
Known by the name of the Odyssey
By the firm of Honda it's manufactured
With it, it's owners seem to be enraptured

But I'm here to tell of a different tale
By which the vehicle does prevail
It seems it's patterned after the hearse
Its preoccupation with funerals seems perverse

Ancient Homer himself told an exciting tale
Of a ten year post war trip in great detail
It was, you'll recall, a trip full of grave travail
After two millennia the name would prevail

But now the name has been purloined
And to a Japanese van it has been joined
I don't think this use Homer intended
It seems to me the name's been upended

Whenever I chance to see an Odyssey
Thoughts of ruination just creep over me
It's simply a matter of the side appearance
That results in vivaciousness interference

I was often told my mildly morose association
Of hearse and Odyssey was my imagination
But then one day, you know, I chanced to disturb
A silver Odyssey at a local funeral parlor's curb

I was certain this juxtaposition was no coincidence
Thought to myself this surely isn't the only incidence
Where the Odyssey and a body shared the same position
Where the qualified driver would best be a mortician

Yes, as I noted before, it is just the side view
That causes the thoughts of death to ensue
When you note the side window configuration
You'll understand, we'll have design correlation

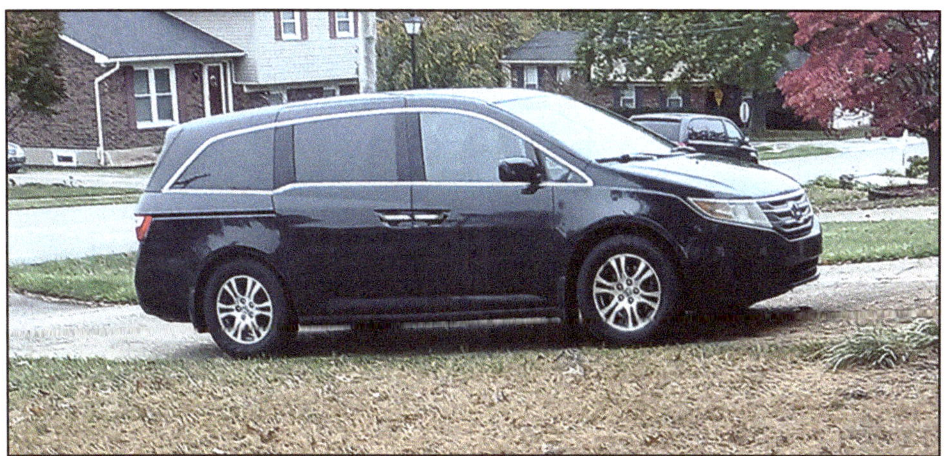

Odyssey

Indiana – The Dark Continent

Lest there be any major misunderstanding
And statutory shortcomings notwithstanding
This work is certainly not a serious critique
But rather is intended as a work tongue in cheek

While it's not my intention to offend
Still I fear I may do so in the end
It's the funny bone I intend to poke
I surely hope Hoosiers can take a joke

It's no coincidence that the name Indiana
Rhymes so well with the dreaded fruit, banana
Located, as it is, just north of Kentucky
That's the only thing about it that's lucky

So now I promise I'll do my level best
To put the ideals of Indiana to the test
By asking about the origin of the toothbrush
Invented elsewhere it would be the teeth brush

Heard that the Kennedy Bridge was made
So Hoosiers could swim south in the shade
I don't know for sure that this plan was true
But it seems no other way to Kentucky would do

For many years it has often been related to me
That things in Indiana simply are not free
You see quite simply beggars can't be Hoosiers
So at least the folks in Indiana aren't all losers

Crime, as you can imagine, is big in the state
So when crime happens Hoosiers call and wait
And who do you imagine they bother to call?
Why the Indianapolis, of course, that's all

Indiana has an Air and Space Museum
I went there expecting a grand coliseum
Was expecting to see an aerial infrastructure
What I found was a completely empty structure

In Indiana the Philharmonic, it seems, is all the rage
They recently doubled the width of the band's stage
With the expansion came a hefty rise in ticket price, you see
The IPS said, "you can't expect twice the band width for free."

The difference between puppies and Hoosier Sports fans
Are significant and reach well beyond simple game plans
The puppies will grow up and eventually stop whining
While the Hoosier remains childlike and never stops pining

I have given you here some Hoosier examples
Of their cultural heritage, you now have samples
Again I hasten to add this evidence is in jest
But now you alone can judge its veracity best

I hope to heaven these jokes aren't too obtuse
Caught up as they are in this rhyming noose
To make them fit into this scheme I fear
Is to make them somewhat less than clear

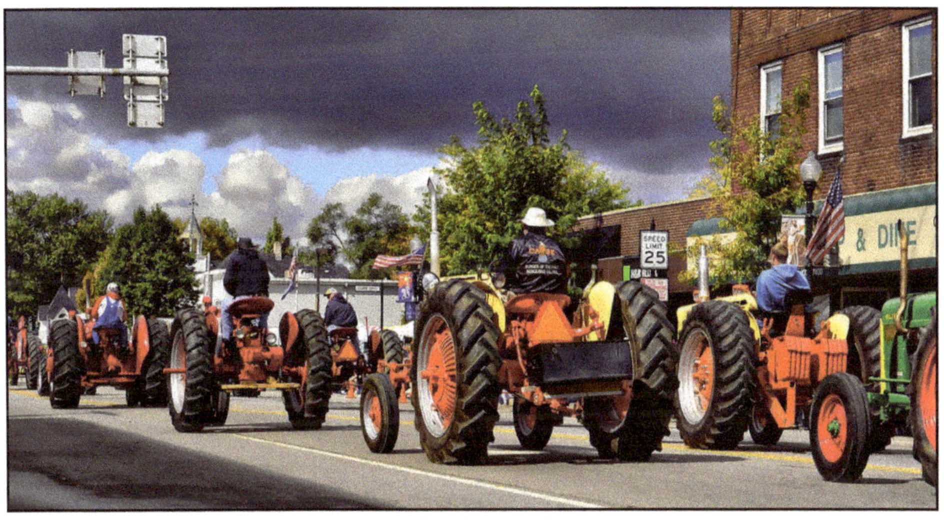

Original Indianapolis 500

In Search of a Topic

This my dear friend is the fourth in a series
Of short piquant poems about things I dislike
Searching for this topic I examined many theories
I'd covered bananas so I thought food I would strike

Started this trip with the baleful banana
Went on a journey in search of the Odyssey
Next I explored the shortfalls of old Indiana
Which led me to consider the topic of geodesy*

But I found nothing to dislike in that scientific branch
So I turned my attention to other topics and situations
I tried to give my imagination complete carte blanche
But decided to avoid more complicated human relations

But what, oh what, should I write about
To what could I bring some thoughtful light
What would make life better if it were left out
Enlightening that, would make the world bright

There would be nothing revealing in covering diseases
And little to add on the topics of war and revolution
See nothing new in pollution and the resulting wheezes
Must contrive a negative that would make a contribution

And suddenly it struck me with a powerful force
The dislike I'd been searching for all this time
It was the search for a topic I hated of course
The search itself was the fodder for my rhyme

Not having a topic remains the ultimate deprivation
It is to be without purpose, to meditate upon nothing
It is to have a whirlwind of thoughts without collation
There's no organizing principle, ideas good-for-nothing

Of course, there are so many sources for topics
Current events as recorded in various news sources
Locations to consider from the poles to the tropics
These, of course, are just a few of myriad resources

But none of these depositories was working for me
I had to find something clearer that hit nearer to home
And then I realized I was looking, but I couldn't see
My struggle for a subject was a search and find syndrome

Yes the source of my discontent was well inside me
I needn't go looking in papers and books for inspiration
Search for an unlikable factor was found by letting things be
The task at hand, in itself, ended the search frustration

*Branch of mathematics dealing with the shape and area of the earth or portions of it

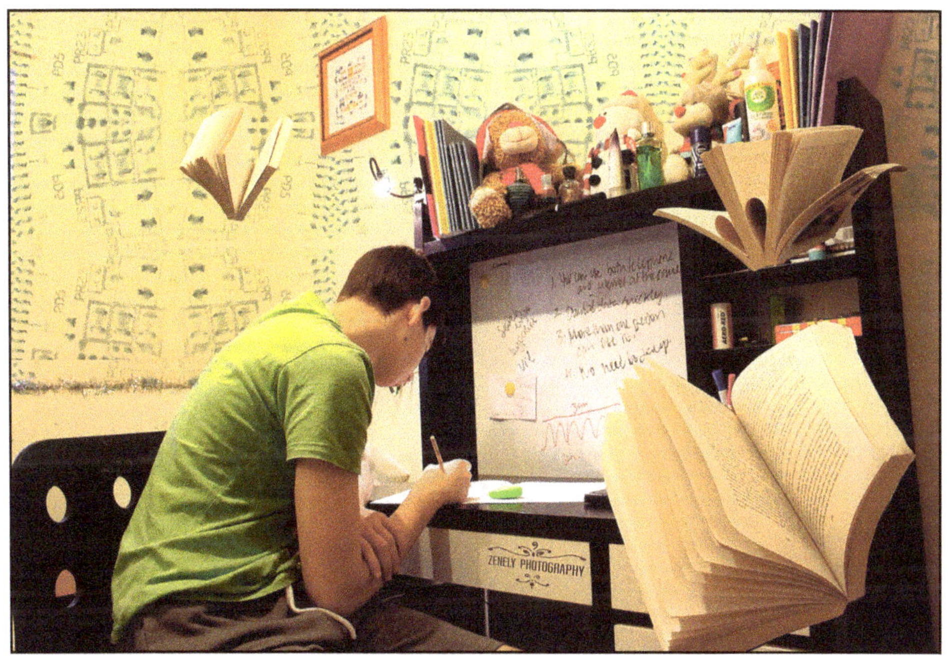

Searching for a Topic

CHAPTER THREE
Likes

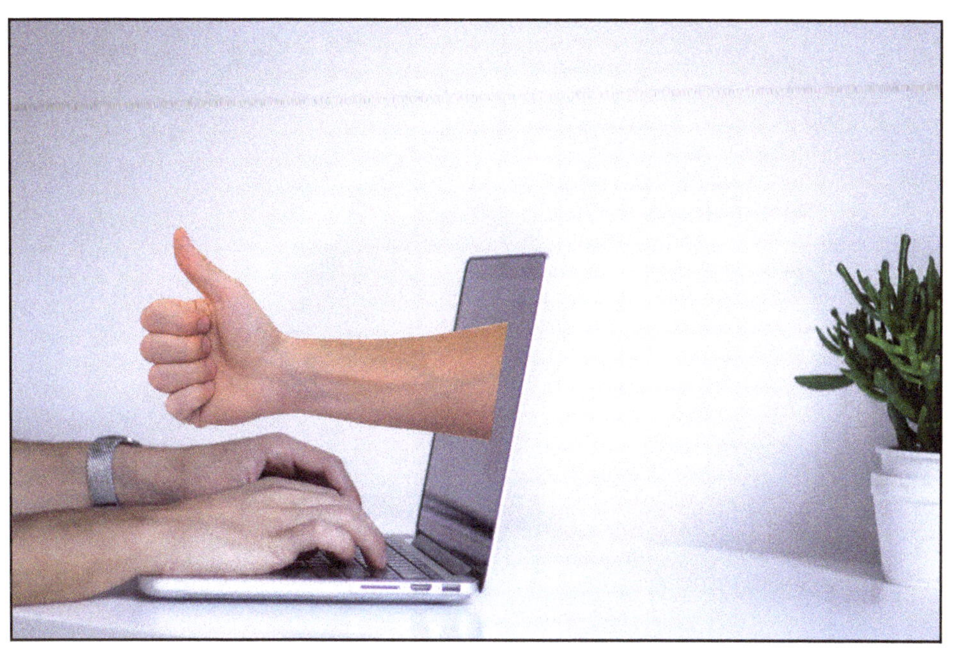

An Opposable Thumb Signaling No Opposition To The Following List

Caramel Carousel

This is the first in a series
Of things that I truly like
Will try to answer your queries
'Bout the good and the bad alike

Caramel is my favorite flavor
It puts plain chocolate to shame
It's the one taste I most favor
Overindulgence is no cause for blame

It makes whatever you put it on taste better
In fact it makes consumption exciting
Just the thought of it makes my mouth water
That's why I'm putting this down in writing

340 degrees is the magic melting point
This is where you get caramel from sugar
Sugar at this temp may burn but won't disappoint
In a dry batch no crystals form in the cooker

In a wet batch things are more controlled
Water prevents burning if added to the mixture
This mix is less likely to burn I am told
But crystallization becomes more of a fixture

Caramel reaches its full potential
When added to other things
It proves itself very essential
When to other sweets it clings

Caramel ice cream for instance
Is a treat that is seldom beat
Caramel on vanilla at my insistence
Even delicious when added to meat

And then there's caramel icing
Tastes great when slathered on cake
It's delicious on other things enticing
I'd lick it off for caramel's sake

I'd best stop here lest I belabor the point
It's obvious caramel is my favorite
King of the flavors it I would appoint
In any application I would savor it

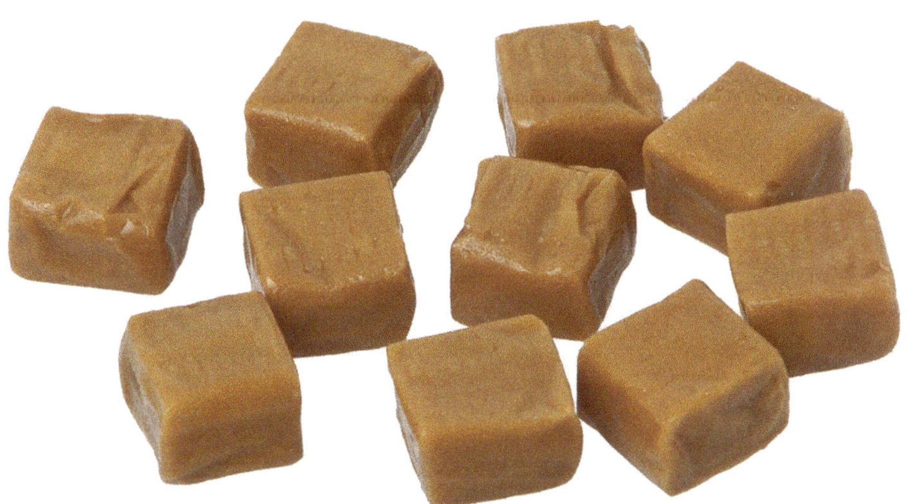

Caramel Collection

Just The Write Word

This is the second in a series of poems
About things, places, and people I like
You can take this particular one verbatim
Cause it's about a verbal miner's strike

You see, when writing rhythmic, rhyming verses
The meaning of a word alone just won't do
The sound, length, and spelling do count
And in the end contribute to lines that are true

Sometimes a homonym that seems wrong
Strikes so much nearer to the implied truth
For example, the 'write" in this work's title
Conveys the right meaning for this verbal sleuth

There, of course, are tools for the poet aplenty
When he goes searching for THE exact word
The thesaurus and the dictionary are but two
Of even greater use to him; syllables he's heard

Sometimes alliteration adds much to the poetic work
Sometimes something sensual is added to the mix
A search may be conducted to avoid a stilted line
The word with the right beginning helps provide the fix

I mention these and other devices
To show the importance of word choices
It makes me happy when I find the right word
It lends beauty and interest to poetic voices

On my very short list of likes
Finding the right word's near top of the list
Because I spend so much effort
Searching for words that will persist

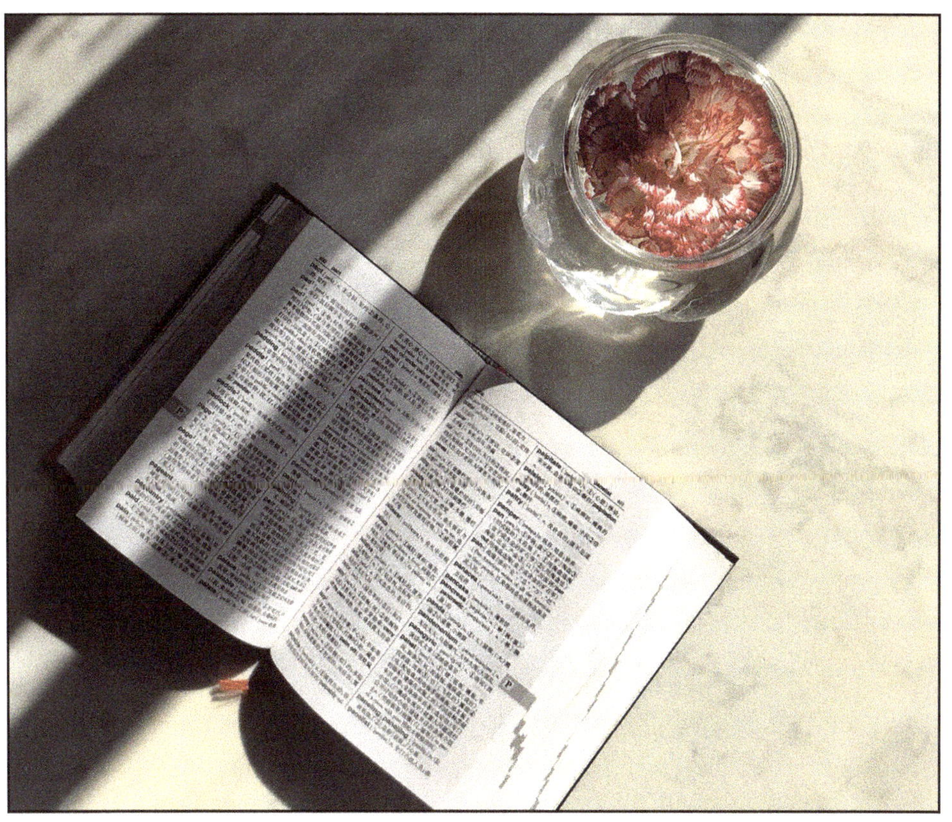

Dictionary

The Test of True Trust

This is the third in a series of things I like
And of all in the series this one's a must
If forced I can do without caramel and linguistics
But I simply can't abide a world without trust

Nothing surpasses the need for confidence
When private thoughts and ideas are exchanged
When two people share their consciousness
Broken trust leads to relationships deranged

I had a relationship, built on unqualified confidence
But I later learned I had misplaced my trust
My thoughts, I believe, were shared to my detriment
My most private inclinations were discussed

As a result of this confidence breach
I lost my most favored friend
Reconciliation it seems is out of reach
Misplaced trust burned me in the end

So you see why well placed trust
Is a thing that I most highly value
Given what misplaced trust cost me
Confidence is a thing I can't overvalue

It's not that I'm ashamed of the thoughts that I shared
In fact, in the proper arena, I would universally share them
It's just that they're confusing without pertinent context
With the unqualified, unvarnished truth I'd compare them

With this confidant I had a good record
At least to date I had never been burned
Breaches were unknown, yet never explored
No, no lack of confidence was ever discerned

But my true love took time to warn me
And I surely took that warning to heart
I shared no more thoughts with the offender
Still those earlier thoughts caused my love to part

I think this is the reason
For my love's demise
False narratives contributing
Would be no surprise

Since the onset of the end of my lover's communication
My resting tremor has quite greatly increased
The complete and total lack of information
Has caused my joy in life to greatly decrease

I have no idea of what was said by who to whom
I only know that I have been cut off from our common room
The results of this painful ostracism is far reaching
I only know that there is no future in beseeching

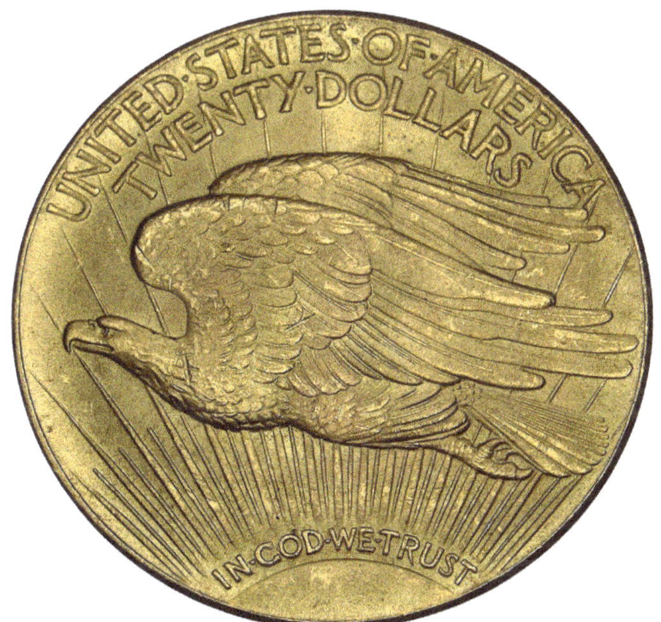

Properly Placed Trust

*Webster's and the O.E.D.**

My favorite book is the dictionary
Tall tales to tell are there
Pneumonoultramicroscopicsilicovolcanoconiosis** is one of them
Stories common and rare

Story lines can be found there with appeal
It can best be seen as a mystery book
Sonorous semantic solutions to reveal
Where verbal vacuums receive a second look

Within its pages many a mystery is solved
The book is a resource most eloquent
By it many a heated argument is resolved
As an authority it is most elegant

As a bonus it provides an etymology
It is replete with information obscure
You can find words like Entomology
The precision of language it helps insure

Info includes identification of part of speech
It helps to insure proper usage
It puts educated grammar within reach
It helps avoid simple abusage

It even provides proper pronunciation
Difficult words it helps you pronounce
It's an aid in basic word enunciation
You get more verbal value per the ounce

It can even serve as a travelogue
On the way to look up a word
You can get distracted, go all agog
And learn of many words absurd

*Oxford English Dictionary

**lung disease caused by the inhalation of very fine silicate or quartz dust, causing inflammation in the lungs

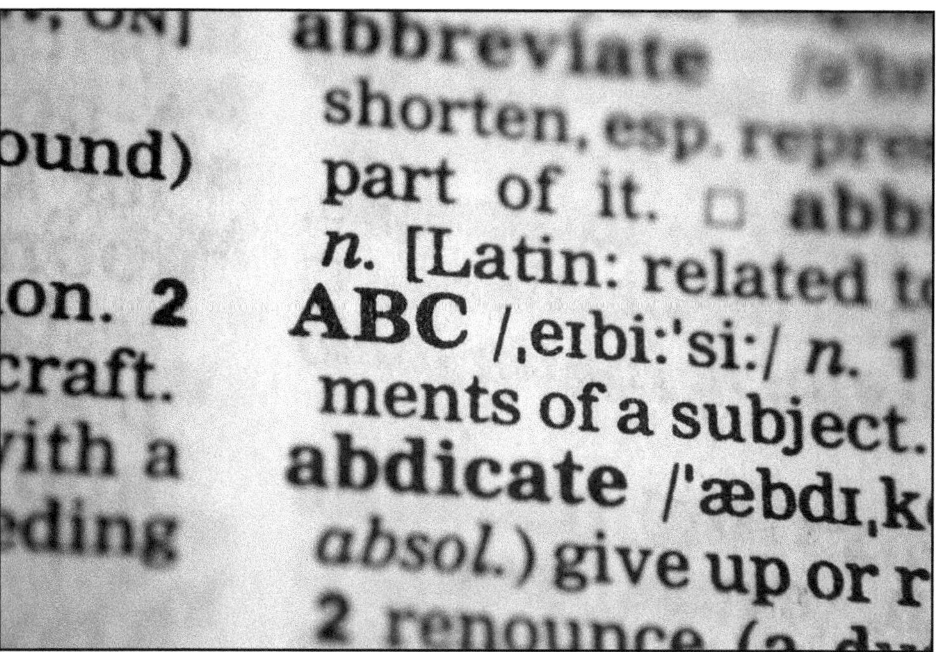

Another Dictionary

CHAPTER FOUR

Disappointments

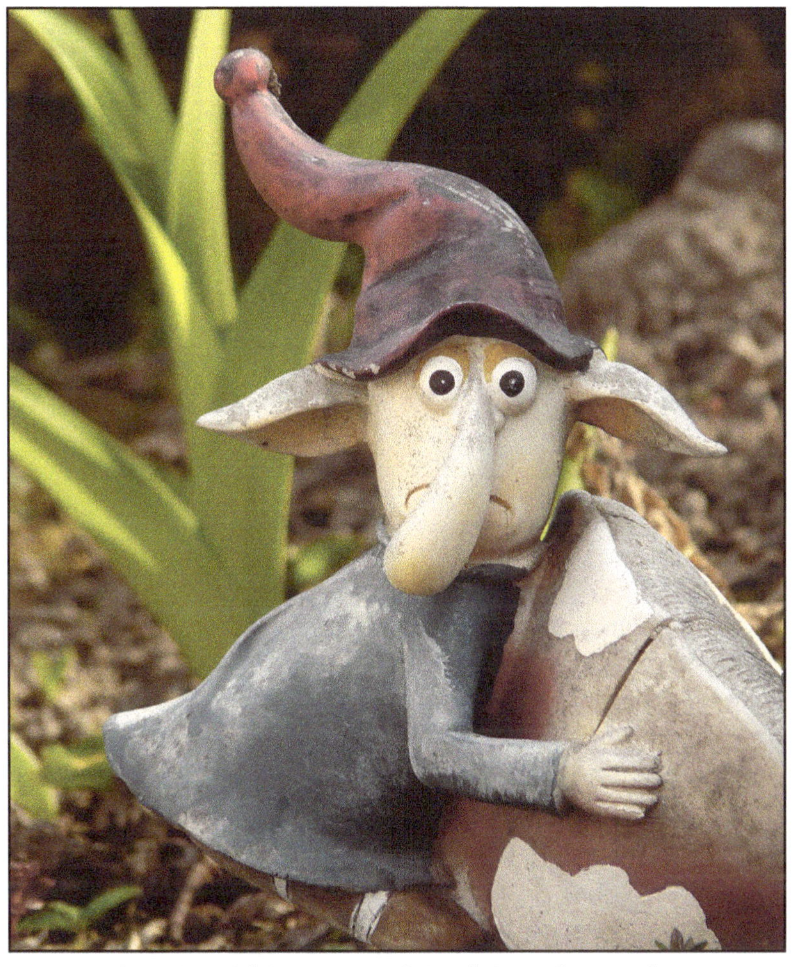

Sometimes Things Just Don't Work Out Like You Plan

Lost Love Lament

Big Brown Eyes
And Long Blonde hair
I'd just fantasize;
I'd see her everywhere

One day I made it real
And drove down to the ocean
All that I could feel
Of love and true devotion

I called the night before
Once I got into town
I could wait no more
I'd see her or I'd drown

She answered with a digital voice
I felt I was defeated
I left a message, had no choice
I felt my soul depleted

I spent the night tossing and turning
I got no sleep at all
In anticipation I was burning
I felt my cold heart start to thaw

Next morning the phone rang
It was her on the line
As I arose my heart sang
I knew all would be fine

We made plans to meet
At a cafe in town
Couldn't wait to greet
Now I wouldn't drown

But once I saw her standing there
I felt an emotional tsunami
No emotion I could spare
As she pressed her spirit on me

We spent the day at the beach
We relived days from our past
So much it seemed was out of reach
I wished this day could last

We drove along the coast
And soaked up all the sun
A day of which I'd boast
We really had some fun

When it came time to go
She told me she had missed me
And then I want you to know
She leaned over and kissed me

When she said goodbye it was no lie
I'd never see her again
I've been searching low and high
But it's like she'd never been

She moved away to another town
A new address she had acquired
Now I can't find her anywhere
What was it she desired?

Did she regret the day we met?
Or was she promised to another?
Was it more than an even bet
She thought I wanted too much of her?

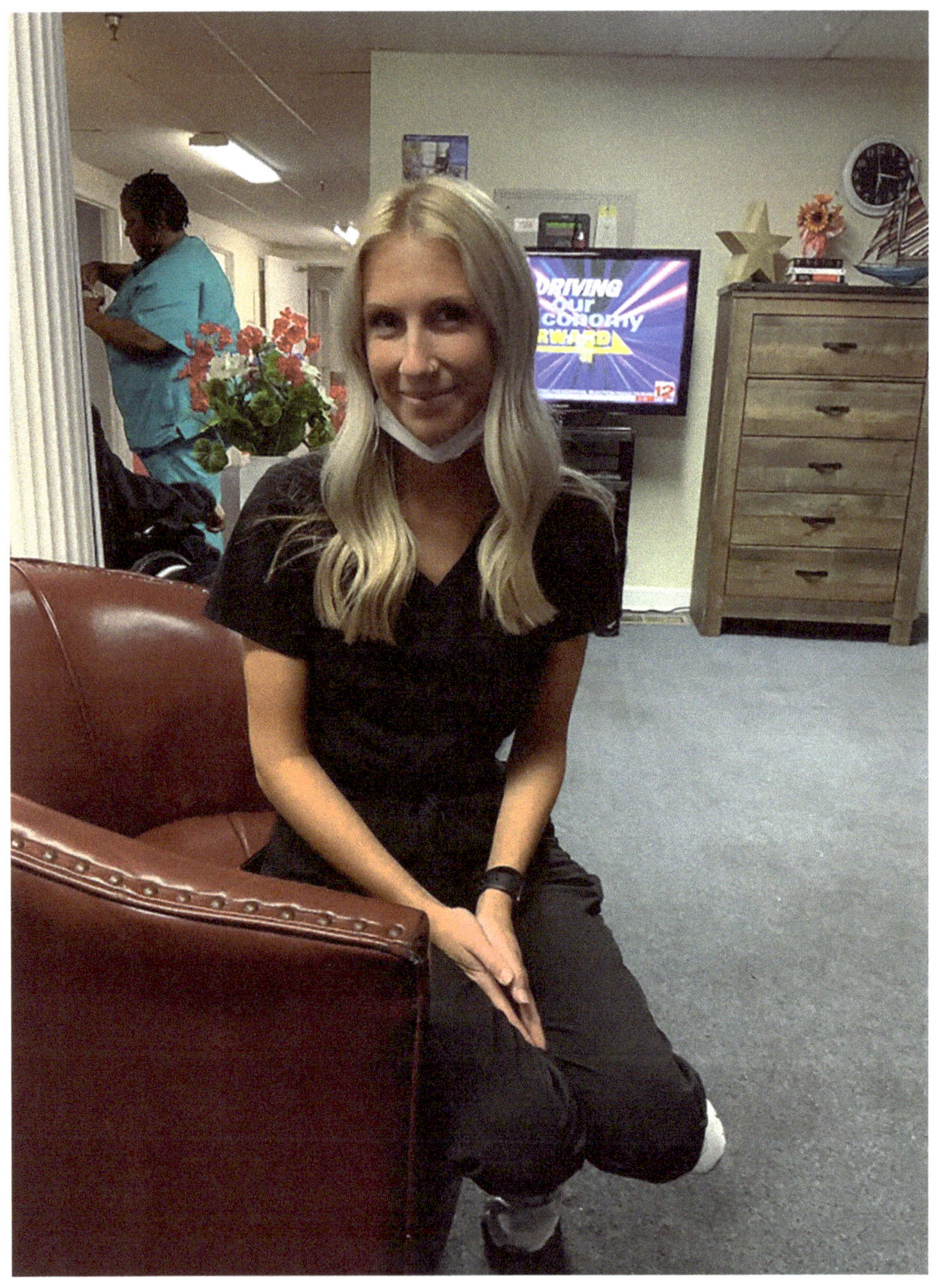

Beautiful Girl, But Not The Subject of The Poem

Joe Smith

A Fool's Errand

I left her there alone on the beach
So much it seemed was out of reach
If I couldn't have her for me
The situation would just have to be

I set out on my trip back home
I never felt so all alone
My memories mulled within my mind
And no real relief could I find

The miles went by as I clutched the wheel
The pain of parting was sharp and real
I fought the urge to turn around
I felt my mood sink slowly down

After some time I arrived at home
The trip was over, no more to roam
I settled in to my old routine
Haunted by what I had seen

The vision of her standing there
The light in her eyes, the sun in her hair
It left me with a passion burning
I felt inside a growing yearning

Two years had passed since I had seen her
Friends knew I missed her by my demeanor
"Well" they said, "why don't you call her?"
"You'll feel better, I'll bet you a dollar"

So I made an attempt, I tried to reach her
To see her again I would beseech her
To answer my call with good effect
And avoid a feeling of utter neglect

The listing I called came from the Web
As I only reached voicemail, joy started to ebb
Still I left a message on the machine anyway
That I had the right party was uncertain that day

The result of the call was no reply at all
I waited for days but got no return call
Maybe my call didn't catch her, I thought
Maybe the list searching had come to naught

Maybe I'd left my message with a stranger
In which case a reply was in little danger
The party I contacted must have gotten a laugh
If I'd reached a stranger and committed a gaffe

But what if I had connected with her
And she didn't reply, decided to defer
Suppose she wanted no contact
There's nothing I could do to add or detract

Either she got the message and decided not to call
Or the message wasn't left on her machine at all
Either way I'd failed to make contact
And it was still true, her company I lacked

Feeling I'd made the right connection
And fearing she had no wish to pursue a resurrection
Of the feelings we had that day on the beach
And again that feeling of all out of reach

Despite all my failures I never lost hope
Even when I reached the end of my rope
I let time go by and prayed for a change
That I waited so long may seem somewhat strange

Now 20 years later, I'm trying again
I turn to the Web, my quest to begin
I have two numbers that match up with my quarry
If neither one is a match I'll sure be sorry

I dial the first and it's out of service
I dial the second, now I'm getting nervous
The second, it seems, is out of service too
I should quit now, but that's not what I do

It's a fool's errand I'm on don't you see
But I can't let her go, can't let her be
If I contact her and she says "No"
Then, and only then, will I let her go

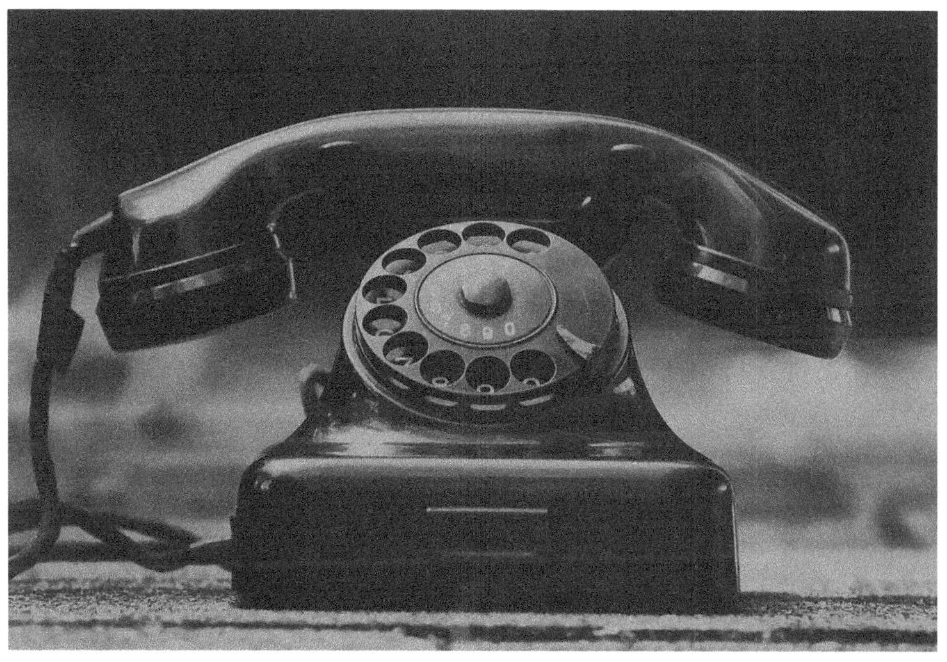

How We Used To Conduct Fool's Errands

On Growing Old

We all age at our own pace
Life's a walk, it's not a race
Some things we gain, some things we lose
Which is which we cannot choose

I thought I'd write about growing old
What I experience and what I've been told
Memories formed tend to fade
You tend to lose friends that you made

As we grow ever older
We grow somewhat bolder
Opinions once hidden
Are no longer forbidden

When you reach a certain age
You hope to be declared a sage
All those things you've always known
That stay with you when you're grown

Memories increase by the score through the years
But memory fades and lack of control leads to fears
That the facts you've collected won't come to mind
And you'll wander through life as if you were blind

Aging is a process full of irony
The more we search the less we see
As we put our memories to the test
We find one fact and forget the rest

The names of old friends filter in
But soon elude us in the end
We try our best to call them back
We try our best, but recall we lack

We think about the places we've been
And ponder what our mind lets in
We relive our past vacations
Forgetting all past altercations

And then there are our several homes
Contemplating each as our mind roams
Celebrations held in each
Events we treasure still in reach

Birthdays, Weddings, and Graduations
Each looms large in our contemplations
Unless of course our memory falters
And leaves us lonely at the event altars

As time goes by our body fails
Our stamina lapses, our constitution rales
Our strength and determination fade
Despite the progress we have made

Loss of friends due to faulty memory
Is not the only loss we see
You see our dear friends pass away
We will too, we know, some day

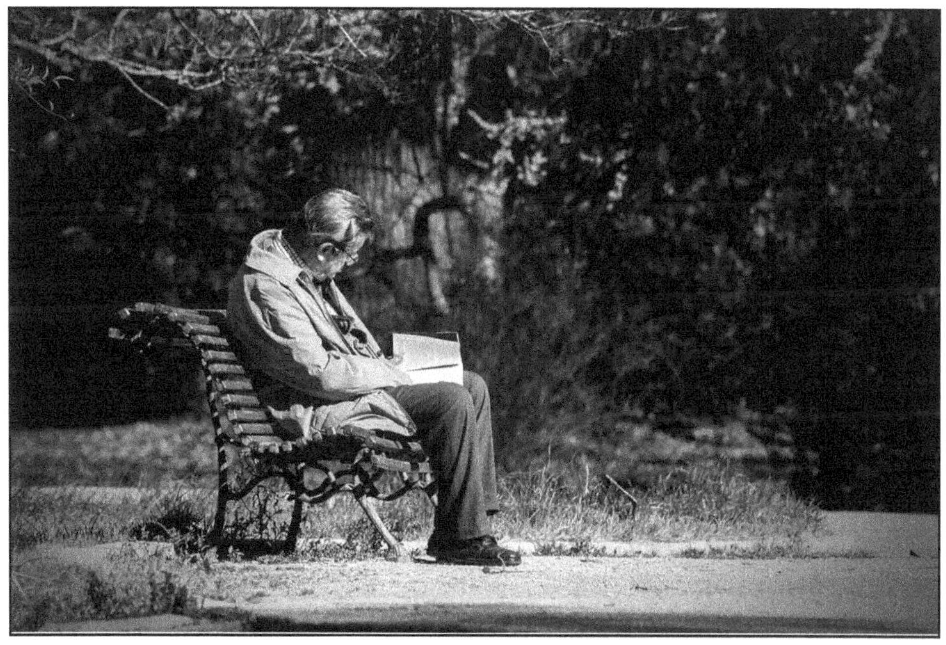

Growing Old Gracefully

Tend My Garden

I planted a garden some six months ago
And everything in it managed to grow
Faces familiar and some barely known
From mere digital seeds faces were grown

I planted my garden along the walls of the hall
And from bottom to top my faces started to crawl
From the left to the right the facial blossoms grew
They grew so in numbers I knew not what to do

Not only faces but animals, common and rare
Raccoons, cats, dogs, and even moths grew there
The garden was filled with family and friends
It was the kind of pictorial garden that love tends

The produce grew rapidly in somewhat unlikely clumps
Nurses, mechanics, and waitresses, some friendly, some grumps
There were therapists, residents, and some care givers too
There was a large group of employees, some old and some new

Over time there were new faces planted
Each face was added, none were supplanted
Digital seedlings were sometimes emailed
Other times the use of the phone selfie prevailed

It appeared that the garden was quite well accepted
But it seems the case that by some it was rejected
On a recent day while I was otherwise occupied
A bad actor, of sorts, a noxious chemical applied

Yes, he / she decided for some reason to spray
The florid faces with a destructive bouquet
Even now I still wonder who was the applier
Despite my suspicions, I'd expect a denier

This wasn't the first time the garden was attacked
The first fusillade was more tightly tracked
The first burst of damage was more narrowly drawn
With minimal damage done with a simple crayon

But this latest attack really set me back
And made me realize there's a feature I lack
It seems I just can't bear to overlook
A personal attack by hook or by crook

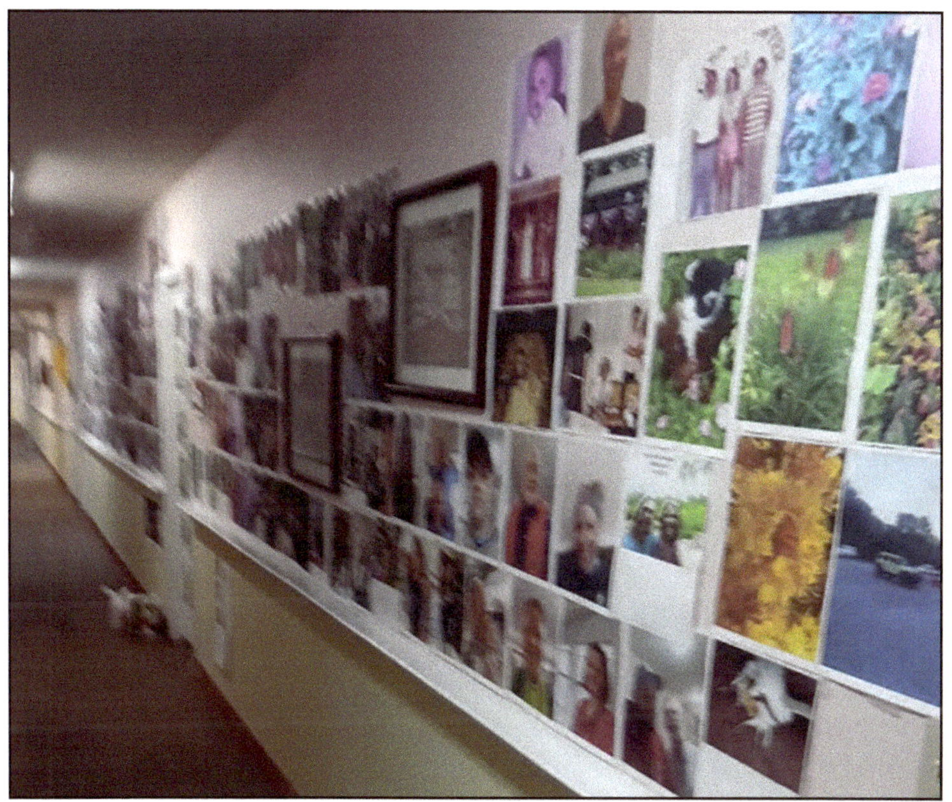

My Garden

Quarantined Again

Again I'm stuck inside this room
I'm not sure how I got here
It has the feeling of a tomb
A room it seems without cheer

There's plenty to do, still I feel trapped
'Cause I can't walk out the door
My energy is all but zapped
Still I continue to pace the floor

I have music and books to appease me
Though they just don't seem sufficient
I need my daily walk to release me
A day without it seems somewhat deficient

Today I listened to some lectures
On Religions of Eastern Tradition
While it led me to some conjectures
They didn't help my condition

I also have some Talking Books
Though the titles don't do it for me
I've given them several looks
But the effect is only to bore me

They bring me my meals thrice daily
So there is no fear that I will starve
But eating alone I don't do gaily
Still from my day this time I will carve

They also bring me my medicine
They bring it four times a day
I take it all, I don't jettison
Or throw a single pill away

I have some aromatic wax
It improves the atmosphere
It comes six tabs to a pack
Makes the place seem less a biosphere

Due to this incarceration
Appointments I have missed
In anxious anticipation
I keep new ones on my list

I'm glad I have my telephone
At least I have some contact
With others on the phone
Though it's their presence that I lack

This is my third Quarantine
You'd think I 'd be used to it by now
All these restrictions I have seen
Just stay calm, no fuss to allow

I'll just sit still for the duration
Take deep breaths and relax
Consider this as incubation
For traits my personality lacks

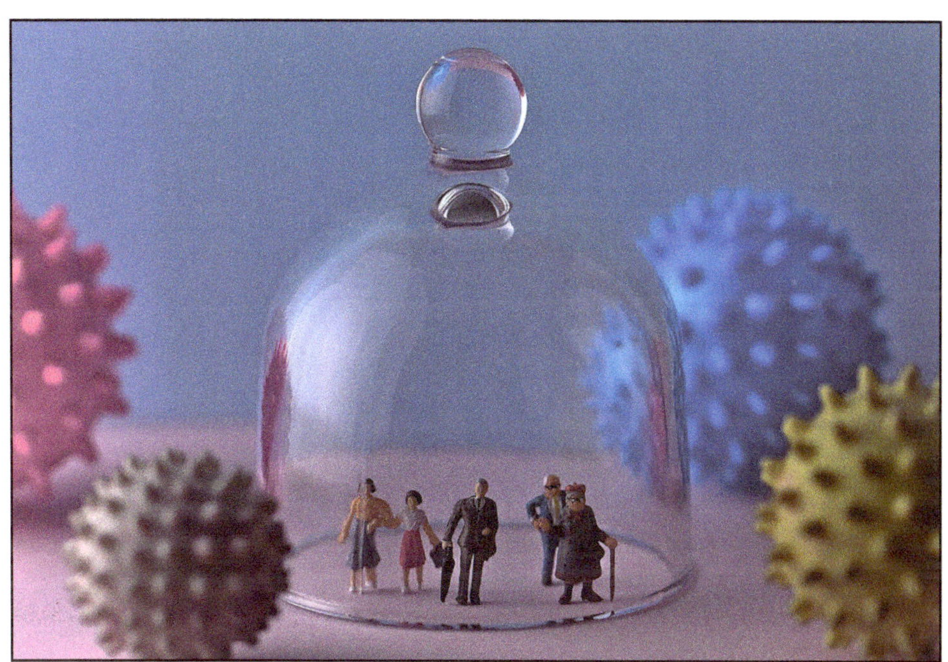

Quarantined Again

No Reply

I've been waiting for an email
Chances are that I will fail
I'm waiting as fast as I can
I'm feeling like an also ran

Why haven't I received a reply
My email was true, I didn't lie
I put a little of me in every line
And yet no response; I'm not fine

I struggled hard to type each line
I tried to write something sublime
Although I didn't quite succeed
I tried my best to fill a basic need

I sent my message with all due dispatch
There may have been an error I didn't catch
This could have been brought to my attention
But instead all I got was reply abstention

So, I'll just sit here 'til something comes through
There's simply not much more that I can do
I guess until I get a reply, I'll just wait
And that's the part of writing that I truly hate

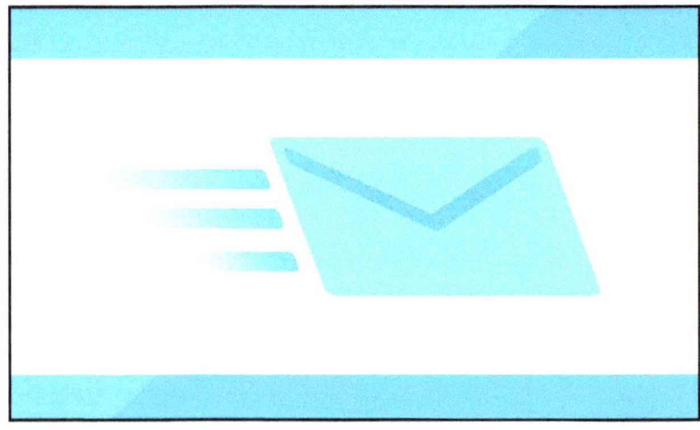

Email

Joe Smith

Alone In A Crowd

There's something I know very well
It's life lived inside a prison cell
It's a simple case of desolation
Lack of contact is its causation

It's like life in a vacant home
Simply sad is this syndrome
No respite from conversation
Internal silence without cessation

It's acting out on an empty stage
Self examination is all the rage
With no audience there to cheer
Simple silence is all you hear

It's a classroom devoid of students
It's care taken beyond what's prudent
To avoid offending the pupils absent
Hope for fellowship is but a fragment

It's the result of those dearly departed
Forced solitude, not for the fainthearted
Recovery, if it comes, takes ages
Re socialization comes in stages

But it's most insidious in a crowd
When essence of spirit is somewhat bowed
Set apart while among one's peers
To be consumed by social fears

There arises a kind of isolation
A layer of self imposed insulation
Wrought of social desperation
Filled full of social consternation

Solitude within a crowd
Makes me want to cry out loud
To be sure I'm not too proud
Hide my distress beneath a shroud

Alone in a crowd's a sad place to be
Solely placed I'm less than free
But to be alone all by myself
Is to just begin to know alone itself

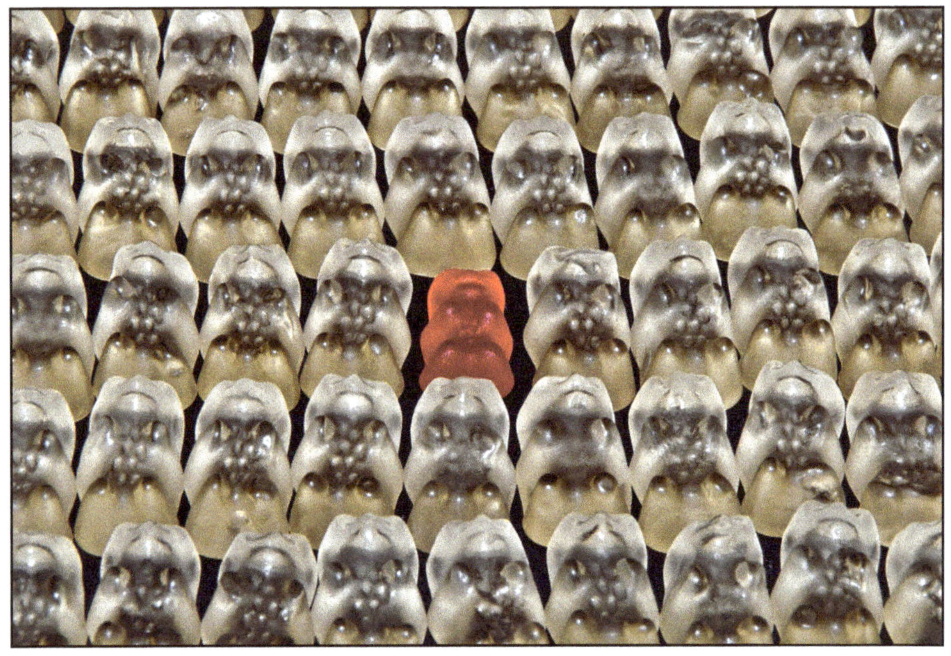

Alone In A Crowd

Joe Smith

The Hedonist's Fright

There are many and various primary sources
Determining these can cost great resources
Among these, of course, are life's chances
Other causes can include chemical imbalances

It can envelope you in a haze
It can last a few, or many days
On your mind it simply lays
It can burn you up in a blaze

It creeps in like a dense fog
Winnie called it the Black Dog
It sometimes robs you of sleep
It can even cause you to weep

It's a tunnel with no light at the end
It's a belief days won't be bright again
It's a black cat with big claws pawing
It's a winter with no hope of thawing

It may even stay with you for years
It becomes the sum of all your fears
It can rob you of all your resources
Dry up all your blood as it courses

It can make you feel guilty, hopeless, or worthless
Most profoundly, it makes you feel mirthless
In the end you may never know what the cause is
You may search all your life and know no bliss

The fact is it may even affect your appetite
Even though you don't understand it quite
Sometimes you simply can't face your food
At times your intake may make you seem rude

Sometimes you simply can't think straight
Your ability to read and write is not great
You simply read and reread to no avail
Your best attempts at composition all fail

Then there's always that great agitation
A feeling of not belonging in your station
There's the risk of the impulsive decision
A risk merely born of your sad condition

Anxiety often comes along with the deal
Worries wind up over the false and the real
Tranquilizers can help to keep you sane
But they really do little to ease your pain

There are also other antidotes for certain
To help prevent the closing of the curtain
There are MAOIs* and lots of alternatives
All solely selected as life preservatives

Sometimes electric shock is called for
Though the thought of it some simply abhor
In truth it's sometimes a solution so elegant
That the choice of it is most intelligent

And, of course, there is psychotherapy
Sometimes augmented by hydrotherapy
Seldom is one approach ever used exclusively
It takes a combination of all conclusively

Resolution depends on the various types to which it conforms
Hedonophobia**, dysphoria***, and dysthymia****, a milder form
You can lose interest in things you used to enjoy
The form it takes helps determine the solution to employ

But you must finally make your choices
Listening carefully to your own voices
Though seemingly conflictive they may be
Your survival my friend, in the end, is key

For when life's light lines are at their lowest
And thoughts slow down to their slowest
Sad solutions begin to become apparent
Expeditious they are, though not inerrant

**Monoamine oxidase inhibitors(MAOIs) were the first type of antidepressant developed.*
*** Hedonophobia is the fear of experiencing pleasure*
****Dysphoria is a state of unease or generalized dissatisfaction with life.*
***** Dysthymia is persistent mild depression*

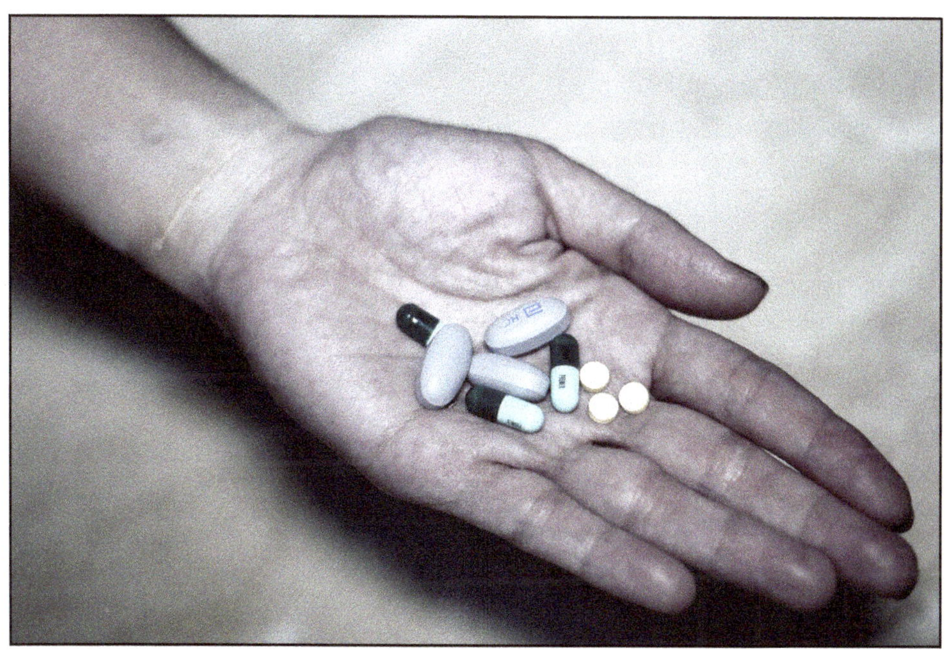

One Antidote To The Hedonist's Fright

Sorry, Not Tonight

It could be an affair of considerable passion
It came about in a rather random fashion
I didn't mean to cause any dissension
No I didn't want to cause anyone tension

There is a woman I've come to know
For whom my feelings have begun to grow
She is a woman with many an obligation
When it comes to duty she's an inspiration

She came to me with a prior commitment
In our relationship it's part of the equipment
It dictates everything we think, do, and say
Heaven knows we both want it this way

Time spent together, of course, is rare and precious
So I'd hoped an evening together would refresh us
But events unforeseen simply got in the way
And pushed off our rendezvous 'til another day

We both of us want to play by the rules
And, of course, abstention desire fuels
There's no future in relationship progression
No point in steps that fuel the obsession

So, it seems, we must remain as we are
And maintain some distance our souls not to scar
But complete alienation just isn't an option
Some Platonic alternative is ripe for adoption

I Think It's Anticipation

I'm not sure of what I'm feeling
But I think it's something real
It's something quite appealing
It just might be love that I feel

I've had a nagging notion
It's gone on for a year or more
That I've imbibed a magic potion
That's brought me to your door

I've kept my own counsel clearly
Have not to another spoken a word
Have chastised myself severely
While total submission I preferred

This love I feel is somewhat tempered
By a slightly anxious component
My joy is somewhat dismembered
By a relaxed feeling opponent

This feeling lends anxiety
To the love I surely feel
It lends a sense of impropriety
To this love I know is real

But it's love in expectation
A less than satisfying thing
It's love in anticipation
That won't let my heart sing

I long to simply hold you
A thing I cannot do
I don't seek to mold you
I want you to be you

I'm in the throes of passion
My heart and mind won't let me be
But there's a wait and see fashion
As I wait to set my love free

Love in anticipation
Is a somewhat cruel sport
It requires inoculation
Satisfaction to purport

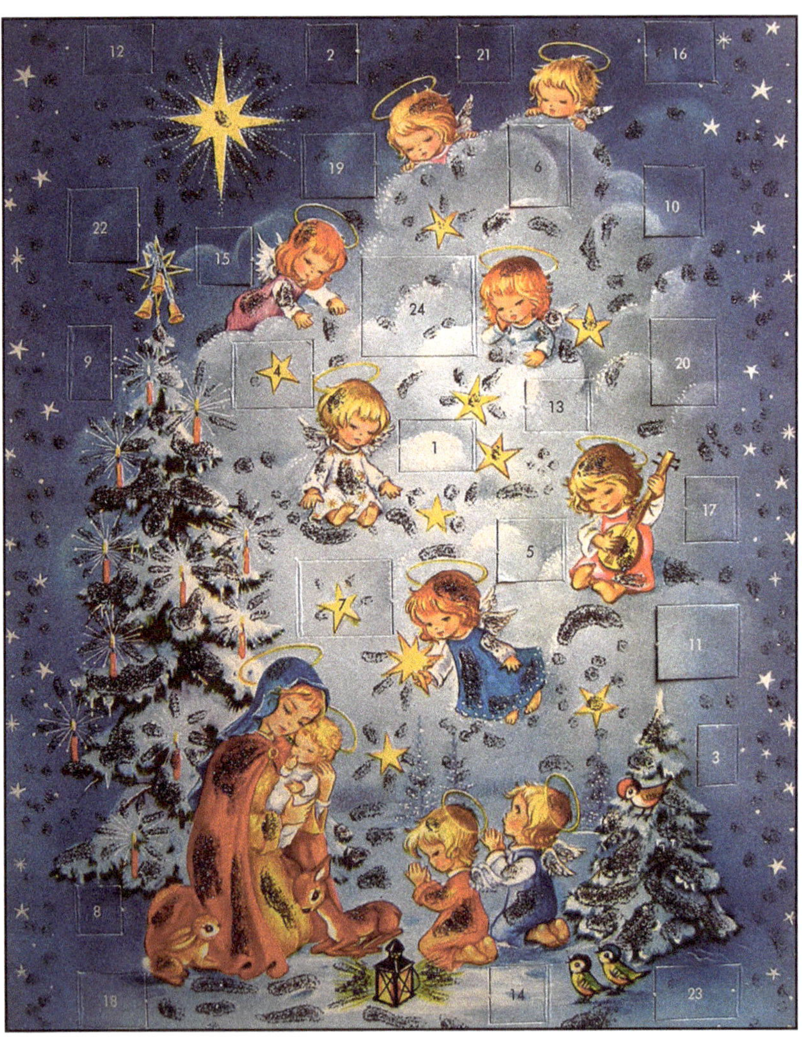

Another Classic Case of Anticipation

Joe Smith

The Fur Lined Trap

I find myself caught in a trap
Of highly unusual construction
All of my energy it will surely sap
And result in my total destruction

To be sure it's of my own making
But no rules I intended breaking
Certain risks I was surely taking
My love thirst I was slaking

The trap is lined with the finest fur
Which conceals tines of rigid steel
While the lining does comfort confer
The pain caused by the tines is real

I carelessly stepped into the trap
Wasn't watching where I was going
My heart and soul went into the gap
Twas something that I wasn't knowing

It all started when I made a declaration
Not knowing that I had no natural right
It was the natural progression of infatuation
Which I had fought off with all of my might

At first all I felt was the fur
A warm and fuzzy feeling
And next thing, all was a blur
I felt the steel, it wasn't appealing

I mentioned that I had no right
To make that love declaration
Surprisingly it soon came to light
A very disturbing revelation

It seems the object of my affection
Was previously promised to another
Though it earlier escaped my detection
Because I wasn't truly aware of her

Now I find myself in a conundrum
Of considerably large proportion
One that I just can't seem to run from
Because of attendant devotion

Yes it is a somewhat sticky situation
And one of considerable import
One of unintentional insinuation
One I unhappily must report

Highest on my list of priorities
Is a desire to avoid causing pain
To involved parties or authorities
Without driving myself insane

The pain of the trap is unbearable
Despite the comfort of the fur
Yes the uncertainty is just terrible
Made worse by my feelings for her

I fear returning to the days pre-declaration
Just might not be as acceptable to her
She may even see it as a negation
Of the affection I first sought to confer

But nothing, no consideration
Will change the way I feel
Despite this desperation
I know my love is real

And now I find I simply yearn
To lose nothing that we once had
To pre-declaration modes to return
To get there without making anyone mad

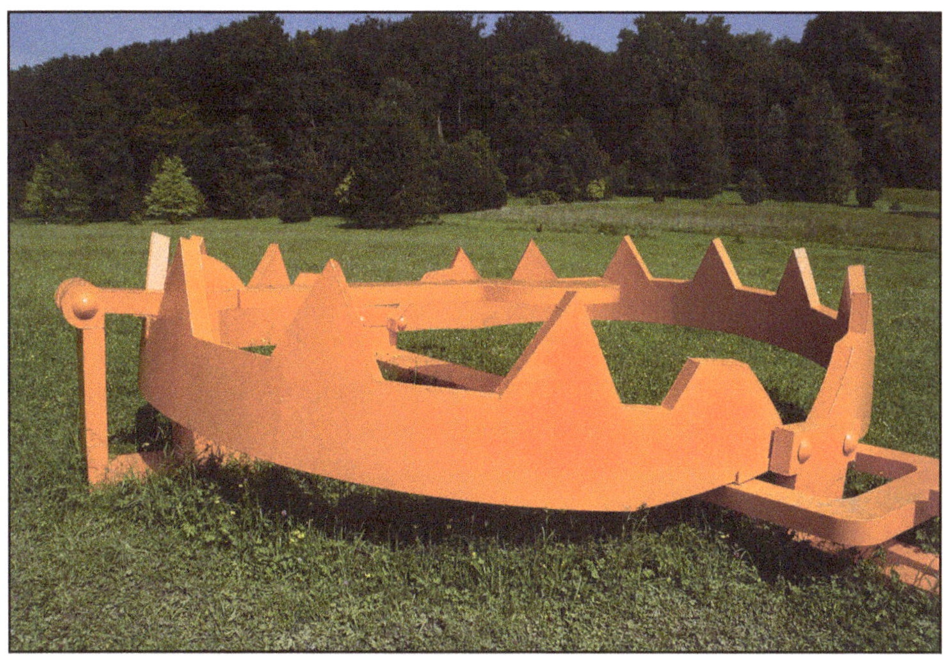

The Trap Stripped Of Its Fur

ECT SOS

Chased by the Black Dog for years
Beleaguered by unnatural fears
He found that he could no longer cope
He felt he'd neared the end of his rope

He'd tried nearly all available medication
To psychotherapy he'd lent full dedication
Many trips were made to psych institutions
To his symptoms were now added delusions

He'd made trips to hospitals out of state
A few that he visited were truly first rate
But for all his effort, things were no better
His mental state was now a psycho fetter

He'd read dozens of books and had gained some insight
But for all that he'd read he still stayed up late at night
Trying to rest without guilt, demons, anguish, and pain
Hoping to learn why he felt so much unearned shame

But as time passed he knew he grew ever closer
To the thought of seeking his permanent closure
With things as they were something had to give
A major change was needed if he was to live

In response to these thoughts of self destruction
And after the multiple failures of medication
There arose the suggestion of electrification
Of the brain so as to improve the situation

Yes, ECT he was told was the solution
To his persistent psycho pollution
"Go ahead", they said "give it a try"
A better choice than to lay down and die

He did some research and then went off to the hospital
He'd progressed through his treatments in a way most logical
Behind him he'd left a host of antidepressants in his wake
He wasn't sure how much more of this distress he could take

He accepted as fact that an induced seizure
Might yield a better life and even some leisure
For he hadn't been able to sleep or rest in awhile
And simply giving up was just not his style

The first night on the ward he rested and dutifully fasted
For general anesthesia was needed for the treatment forecasted
He was up early the next day and he donned two flannel gowns
Then he sat on the bed and waited for the Doc to make rounds

The doctor stopped by and explained the procedure
That memory loss could result was the only feature
That caused him to have any concern or misgivings
Then he thought, this is how these Docs make their livings

And so then and there he decided to give it a go
Despite the fact that there was much he didn't know
The step he would take was highly recommended
By his closest friend whom he would not have offended

It was this recommendation so recently given
That brought him to this point, by it he was driven
So he proceeded into the lab and lay on a gurney
He was secured with straps to ensure a safe journey

Next electrodes were affixed to his head
He reminded himself, "there's nothing to dread"
The anesthetist then started the slow drip
To ensure him a safe and painless trip

When he awoke it was as if nothing at all had transpired
The only effect he could detect was the headache he'd acquired
It wasn't until later he found memory loss and confusion
Were byproducts of this electro-convulsive intrusion

He experienced twelve of these procedures
Over a four week period he had all these seizures
In the hospital, you see, time slowly passes
Like an hourglass charged with molasses

They say the proof's in the pudding
By that measure, results were off putting
He found that little enough had changed
And that little more had been gained

His friend said she noticed a difference
She didn't say "better" out of deference
Because he truly felt not a bit better
Despite following directions to the letter

For many ECT is just the ticket
A way out of the psycho thicket
It produces many success stories
For those willing to mine in its quarries

But as for our friend here it was simply a bust
More treatments were suggested and I trust
That you understand why he declined them
The lack of success he needn't remind them

And so after his release he continued to search
For an answer that wouldn't leave him in the lurch
And later, in a new method, he thought he had found it
But FDA approval was pending and regulations bound it

Eventually the new method was given the green light
A device came on the market to the manufacturer's delight
He followed the development of the device play by play
And the result of those efforts is a tale for another day

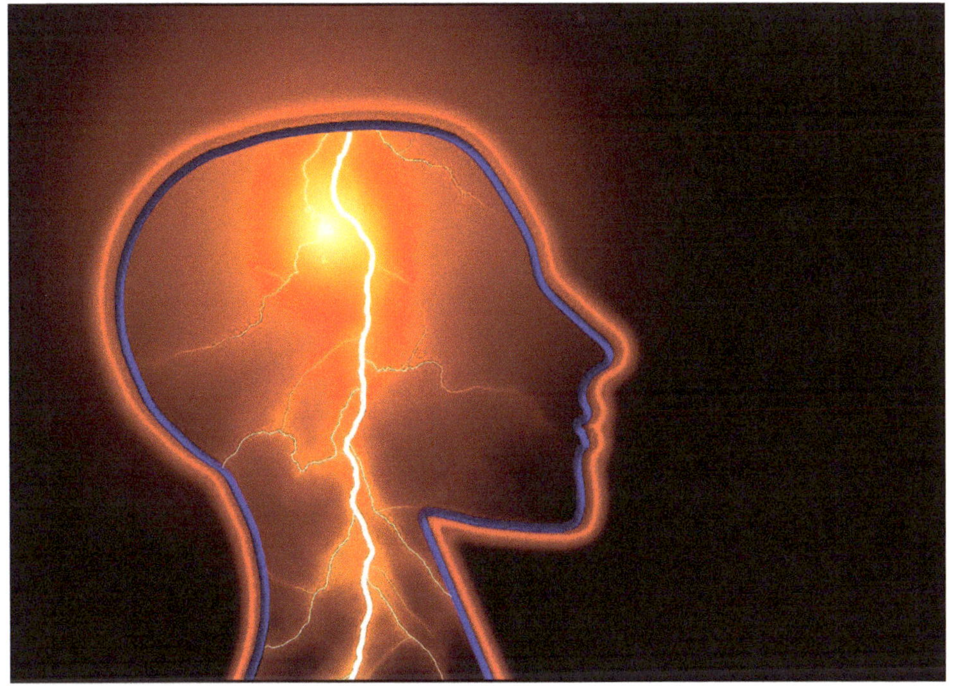

Electrically Induced Seizure

Requiem for a Relationship

I don't think I can remember
When I have been so sad
Our friendship, it seems, is dying
Not knowing why is driving me mad

Been so long since I have held you
Felt your warmth within my arms
I fear I cannot live without you
I miss you and all your charms

Don't know what has happened
To make you stay away
I fear I have offended you
Made you feel you couldn't stay

I've tried my best to maneuver
Within the boundaries that exist
Tried to follow all the rules
To help our relationship persist

But I fear something has happened
To gum up the delicate works
Something untoward has arisen
And in the background lurks

There's a reason you won't tell me
Just what I have done wrong
Yes, some reason to repel me
Despite an attraction that is strong

I'm really at a loss
I don't know what to do
I still don't know the cause
I've never been this blue

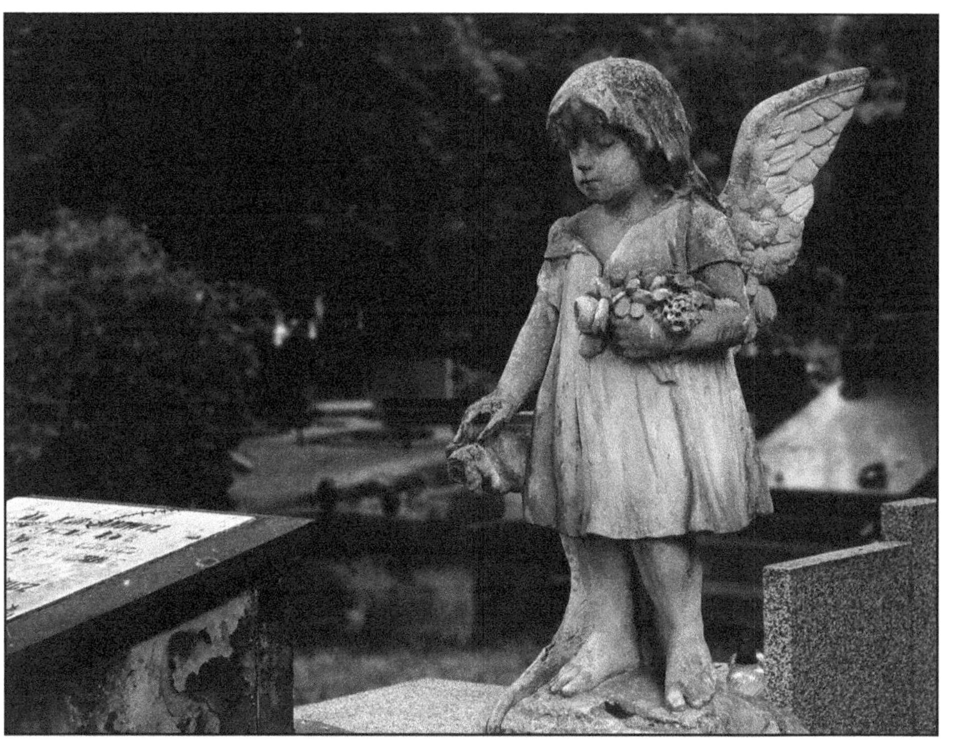

The End of the Relationship

The Loss of Our Managing Therapist

This is a tale of Lisa Anthony
Whose loss is causing me agony
Though she is but one of many
Of her equal there is not any

I will assert without any guile
Most missed will be her smile
When she smiles she uses her whole face
With it pain and frustration she does displace

I mean to say that she smiles with her eyes
Her lips alone her mood can't disguise
When she enters a room it lights up
The dreariest day she will spice up

I know this because I've been in her charge
And it surely was her smile by and large
That brought me each day encouragement
And warded off the bane of discouragement

It doesn't hurt that Lisa is beautiful
It made it easy to behave and be dutiful
I found it easy to follow her instructions
Was never offended by her many corrections

To say I'll miss her would be an understatement
To fail to state this would constitute a misstatement
My fervent prayer is that she'll soon return
But this of course is a matter of self-concern

I know Lisa has other obligations
She occupies many other stations
It's selfish to want to detain her
I wouldn't want to restrain her

But I know I surely will miss her
No way I could ever dismiss her
Despite my selfishness I hope to soon see her
But in all fairness I know I must free her

So in closing I'll wish her good luck
Though on her it's easy to get stuck
I'll just have to grit my teeth and let go
And be happy she's someone I got to know

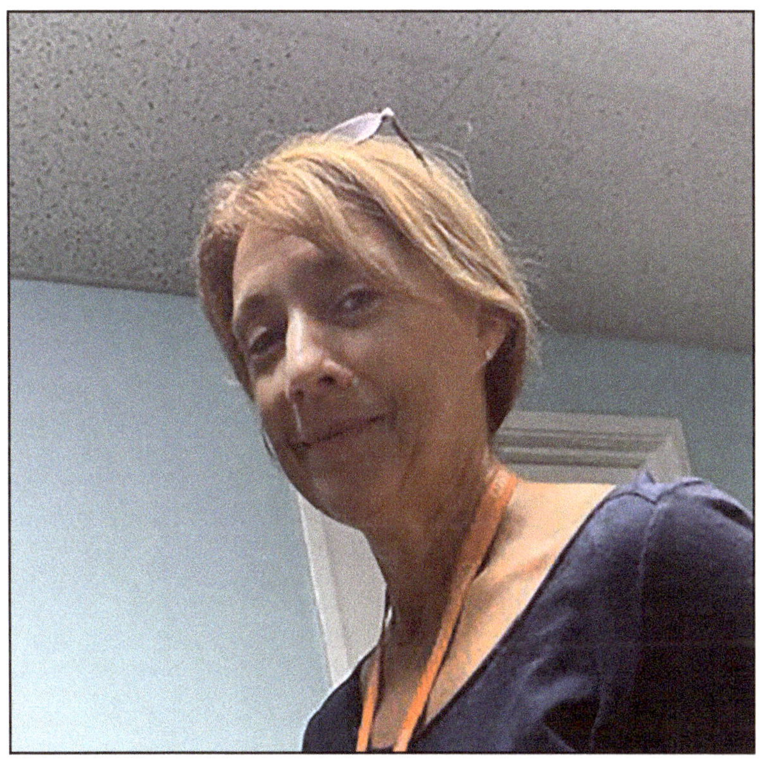

Lisa Anthony

"You Can't Go Home Again"

This is a story of unusual action
A tale of decided dissatisfaction

It is a tale of just not belonging
A tale of near constant longing

It's simply a tale of not quite knowing
Where one belongs or where one is going

The protagonist at one point left his home
And throughout this nation he had to roam

He spent four years out on the West Coast
Of his time there he often would boast

Next he packed up his family and moved to the East Coast
Soon after arriving he decided he liked the West most

He eventually settled on a mountain in Tennessee
This, it seems, was the one place he wanted to be

But living there left him with a longing
At times he had a sense of not belonging

From time to time he would start pining
For his family home, he would start whining

And then to add insult to his discontent
A visit to his family home lent a lament

To his rapidly growing dissatisfaction
With his place in the world and his reaction

It seems when he went home he missed his friends
From the Tennessee residence which security lends

He finally decided to take some action
And so he prayed for bi-location satisfaction

He recognized that he had two homes
Fortunate case for he who often roams

But for now he can't go home again
For he isn't sure just where to begin

Location in either makes him yearn
For the other place, his emotions burn

For a more settled mind, two homes possessed
Would be a blessing, of that he's confessed

But for now he'll seek satisfaction
In the individual site's attraction

In short he will simply do his best to endeavor
To seek satisfaction in the locale whichever

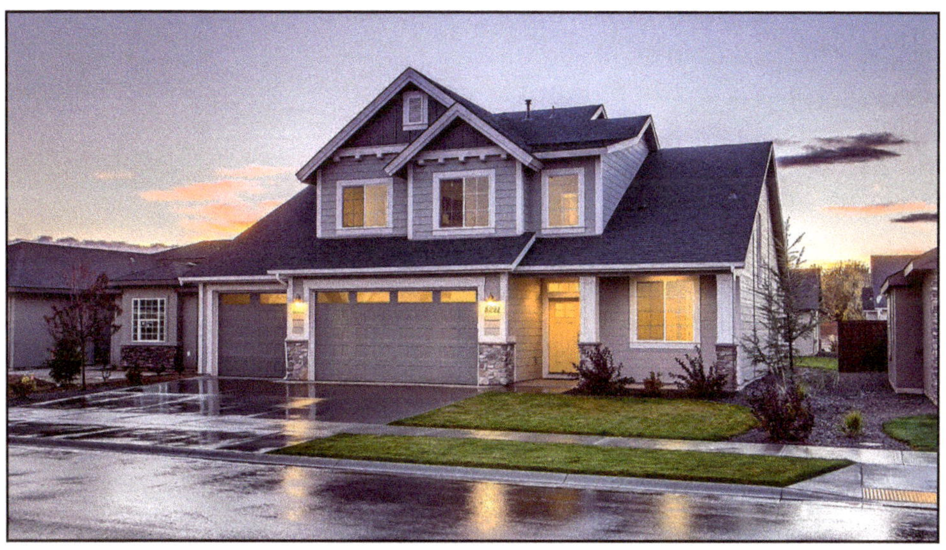

A Home

Shutout

Sometimes I'm left with a sense of longing
There's a definite feeling of not belonging
Sometimes I'm left with a nagging doubt
'Cause from a social group I've been left out

I had that feeling a short while ago
When I was rejected by a friend I know
I expected to be let into the group
But wasn't; it threw me for a loop

I certainly felt I'd paid my dues
And thought that, that dues I'd use
But I was stopped short at the door
It did no good for me to implore

So I went back home and there I waited
Feeling more than a little lost and deflated
With a strong connection to the group leader
I thought that later I would get to meet her

But while I waited I began to sweat
I surely thought I had an in and yet
I decided on a nap as I continued to wait
When I awoke I wasn't feeling so great

I went to where the evidence lay
Out in the lot in a parking bay
There I saw her car was gone
From my grasp she had withdrawn

She started out so safe and warm
I'd vowed to me she'd come to no harm
And now from me she was, again, gone
So I try hard not to fret, but to carry on

I've woven cloth of considerable passion
To sew a uniform of a specific fashion
In order that I might join an exclusive club
That won't induct me and that's the rub

Once again I've been cut out
Of a club I'd rather be about
Love comes close then fades away
Will it return to me another day?

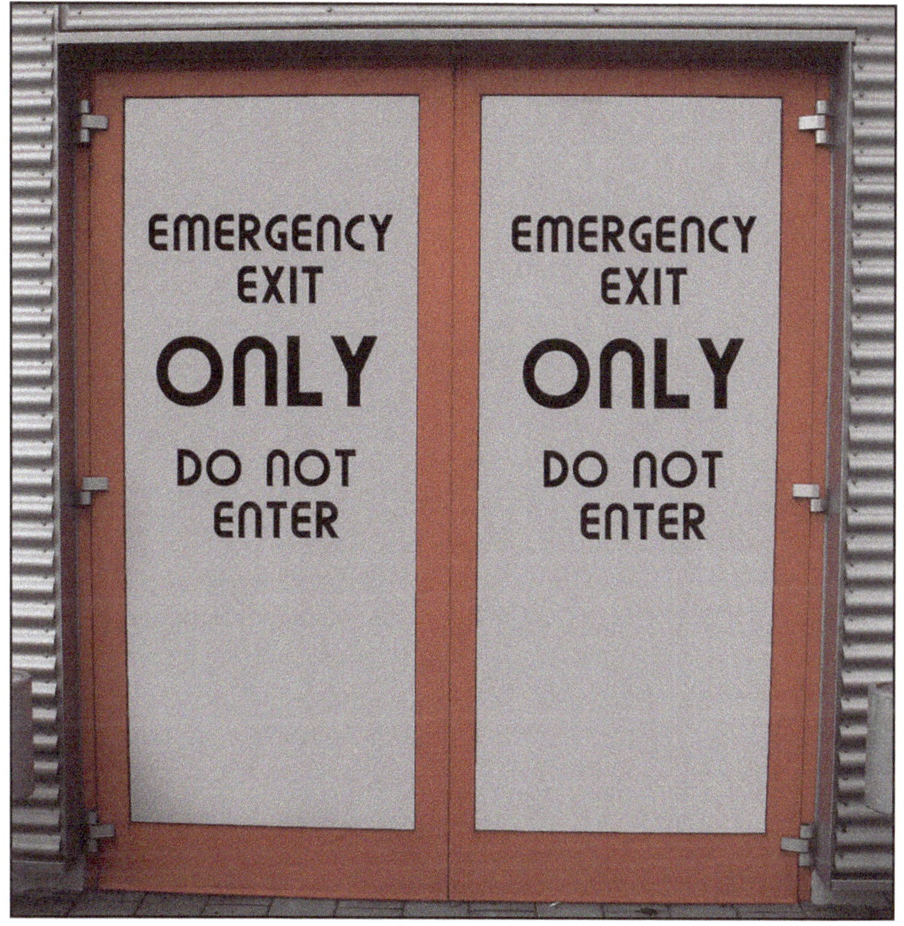

A Shutout Example

CHAPTER FIVE
Poetic Effort

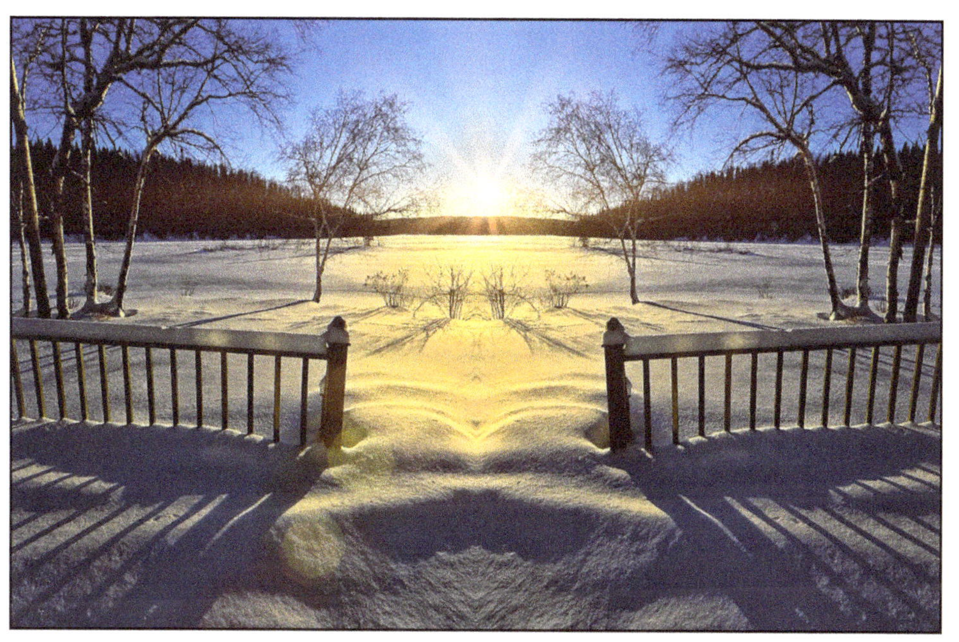

I Wonder if You Can See The Pattern That Is Clear to Me

An Ekphrastic Attempt*
or
*The T-Rex** and His Thesaurus*

Ekphrastic poetry is something I learned about
While engaging in some self education
I just couldn't wait to at least try it out
Actual or Notional, the point is edification

I'll have to try notional as I have no artwork before me
I'll imagine a Tyrannosaurus reading a thick Thesaurus
This seems exciting to me, little chance that it will bore me
When I'm done I hope we can see the great T-Rex before us

I imagine, like me, the beast is into self discovery
He'd use the book as a guide to self enlightenment
He'd look up words reported in notes of his recovery
Trying at length to show signs of his own refinement

Lacking in the social graces
The monster seeks pleasant phrases
Seeking now to change places
With a beast that garners praises

As we gaze upon this wondrous site
We begin to imagine the entries
That our studious T Rex might cite
From current days or old memories

I'm guessing among his first searches
Would be one for the word "extinct"
He'd try this before "pterodactyl perches"
Synonyms for this would seem to be succinct

Next he might search for words similar to "predator"
Interested in finding a polite word to describe his diet
For those who think him a "scavenger" he'd search some more
Frantic to find a civilized explanation rather than to try it

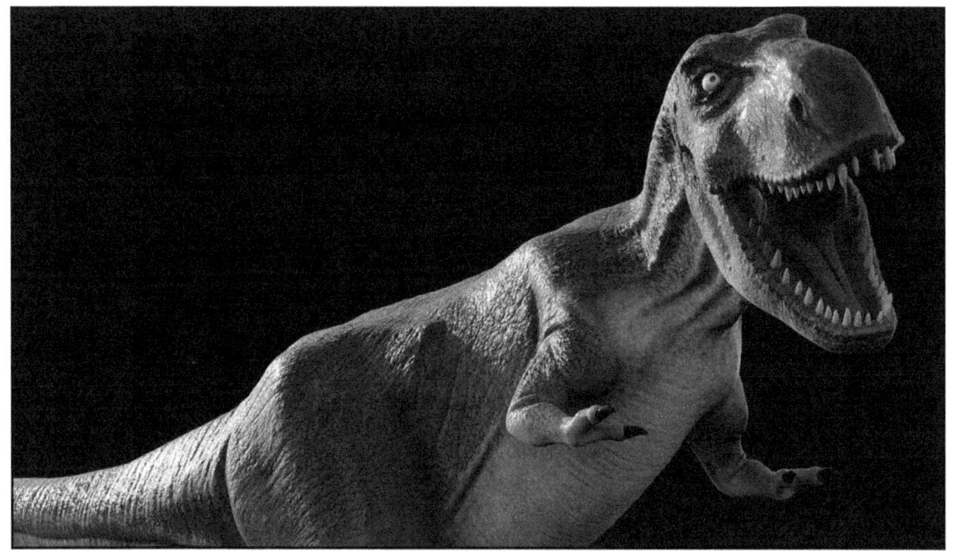

Tyrannosaurus Rex

And then, in his self indulgence, he might look up "regal"
For as we all know he was the king of the giant lizards
Even if hunting provided his sustenance, it wasn't illegal
Dead or alive he would have enjoyed some tasty gizzards

Another word for which he'd search
Would of course be "paleontologist"
For these are the folks whose research
Comes closest to that of a zoologist

And next he'd go on to "leviathan"
For he was known to reach 40 feet long
Of course he'd carefully peruse the text
No chance he'd select a word wrong

Feeling now somewhat more insecure
He searches words of competition
He looks up "gigantosaurus", so obscure
Remaining king is his main ambition

And so trying again to finally fit in
He searches for a word of justification
Seeking a throne for him to sit in
Allowing him rule over an entire nation

A final search might be for "Divine Right"
He'd come up perhaps with "Dominion Theology"
And if, indeed, he did not understand it quite
He might give up and rely more on mythology

**Ekphrastic poetry is poetry written about a work of art, either a real piece = Actual Ekphrasis or an imagined work of art = Notional Ekphrasis*

NB Keats's Ode On A Grecian Urn *is a classic Ekphrastic Poem*

***The REX in T-Rex, of course, means king*

Joe Smith

Brainstorm

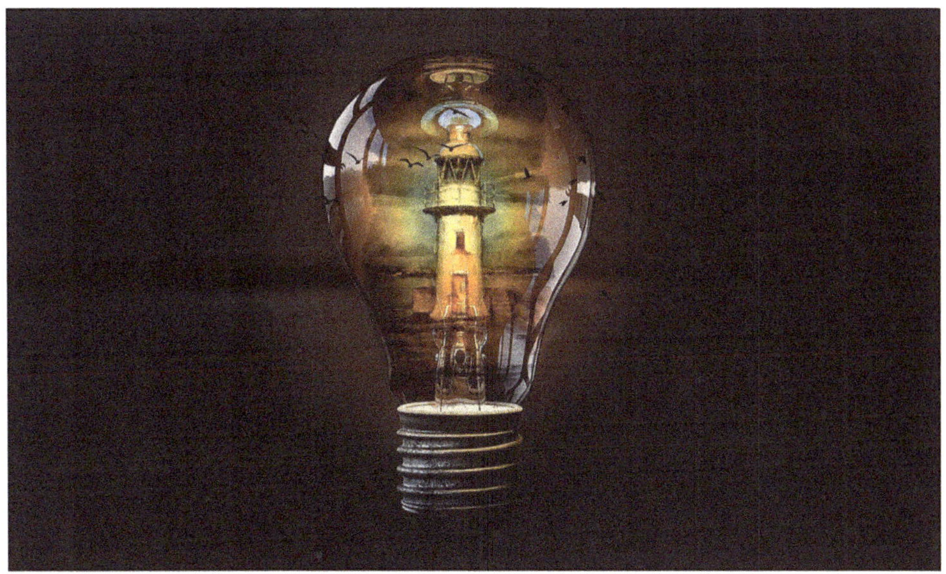

A Brainstorming Innovation

To make something
Out of nothing
That's the plan
Of the poetry slam

I want to write right, right now,
What will be well written and how?
Will it be written well now?

Does it matter the time of day?
We know it did for Hemingway

Get up early in the morning
Before the day is dawning?
Or wait until the evening
When the daylight's leaving?

Should I write alone?
On and on I drone

Does it really matter?
All this mindless chatter

Prayer for inspiration
Prevents incineration
Of strangulated attempts
That sheer effort exempts

Search for relevance
Results in dreadfulness
Generates detritus
Form of mental mephitis*

Close examination
Leads to observation
Of the obvious
To the audience

The offal from the poetic process
Tend to make one somewhat nauseous
But once sound syllables are secreted
The offending ones can be deleted

Something strong, sensible, and true
Is among the best to do
If you can you add emotion
To the positive perceived notion

And finally you have some verses
Some of which life rehearses
Others produced inside the mind
And thereby you escape the bind

**foul smelling gas or vapor*

Joe Smith

Why I Write Poems

Sometimes I wonder
Why I write at all
When so often I blunder
When so often I fall
Short of my intention
At least that's how it seems
Too often to mention
Despite the various themes
I've written some verses
In the past don't you see
About topics like nurses
But there's no guarantee
That they'll like my verses
I guess I write them for me
Though self esteem reverses
Still, though, I let others see
Some let me drain my emotion
Others let me take a position
Some are devices of my devotion
Others help express my disposition
Poems help me think more critically
They take an inordinate amount of time
They require considerable effort typically
Word choice must fit the pattern of rhyme
Sometimes it's fun to play with words
Sometimes I will employ them
Like birds and bugs and bees
With alliteration I enjoy them
And so poems are an exercise
In words and convoluted thoughts
My inner demons to exorcise
In positives and naughts
Though poems needn't rhyme
And there's a thing they call free verse
Mine do all the time

Without rhyme they'd be worse
I try to write what's true
Each and every time
There's only so much I can do
Within the realm of rhyme
I do my best to illustrate
Within these cryptic lines
I try hard not to obfuscate
The truth my word defines
Sometimes I feel compelled
To share the lines I write
My reluctance is dispelled
When I push beyond the trite
And delve into the deep
And dusty corners of my mind
The place I always keep
Those things of which I'm blind
Writing poems helps me reclaim
Those things that I've forgotten
Some of which may defame
And make me feel quite rotten
Others, though, may make me glow
And make me feel ecstatic
Make me happy even though
My behavior was erratic
To share my poems is somewhat bold
Others may not want to see them
But to hide them away I am told
Is to risk that I will be them
That is to say, in some small way
To hide them is to relive them
So the advantages I will weigh
To instead just go out and give them
And so I let my feelings out
And publish my poor poems
And let them know that I can shout
About the ones I show them

In sharing them I feel
Somehow quite retarded
But they in fact are real
So I feel much less guarded
And so this work will end
It can go on no more
Nothing left to append
I hope it's not a bore

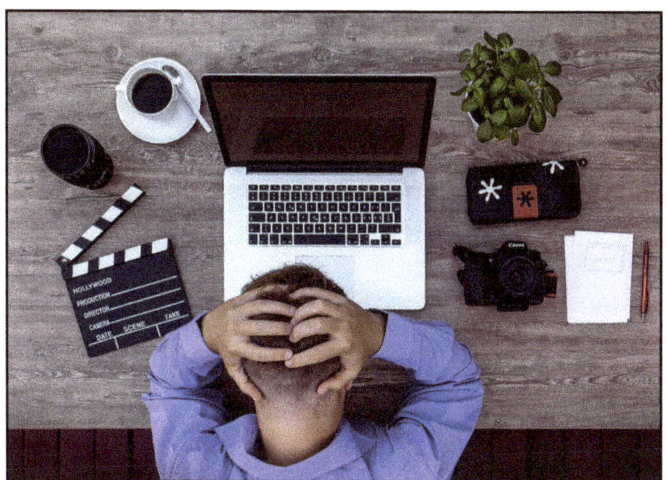

Composition

My Verbal Photos

I wonder if I should let them see
These pictures of inside of me
Or are these all too self conscious
Reflections of my own subconscious

Would they feel that I'm imposing
So much of myself I'm disclosing
All of it enshrouded in code
A safer way for me to unload

To circulate these seems so selfish
Why do I do it, for what do I wish
I think I need some confirmation
About my position in this situation

It may seem somewhat egotistical
To consider these lines somewhat mystical
Of course it's true they don't have to read them
They don't need, but I do need them

If read with some perseverance
They'd see into my transference
Just random thoughts forced into rhymes
Most of them mined from unhappier times

I wonder if I should sift them
Discarding those with secrets in them
Some just state facts but still they seem mean
It's the feeling behind them I hope they'll glean

I hope that they will realize
That these are just an exercise
To keep the dreaded blues away
Despite the things that they may say

This is another way to employ them
I certainly hope they will enjoy them
I hope that some don't bring them down
Cause them to twitch or form a frown

I don't understand the need to share them
Why I cannot just compare them
With the ones I write right now
Some need for approval that they can endow

So here they are for your approval
Or maybe here for your refusal
I hope their meaning you can fathom
As you work your way through this word album

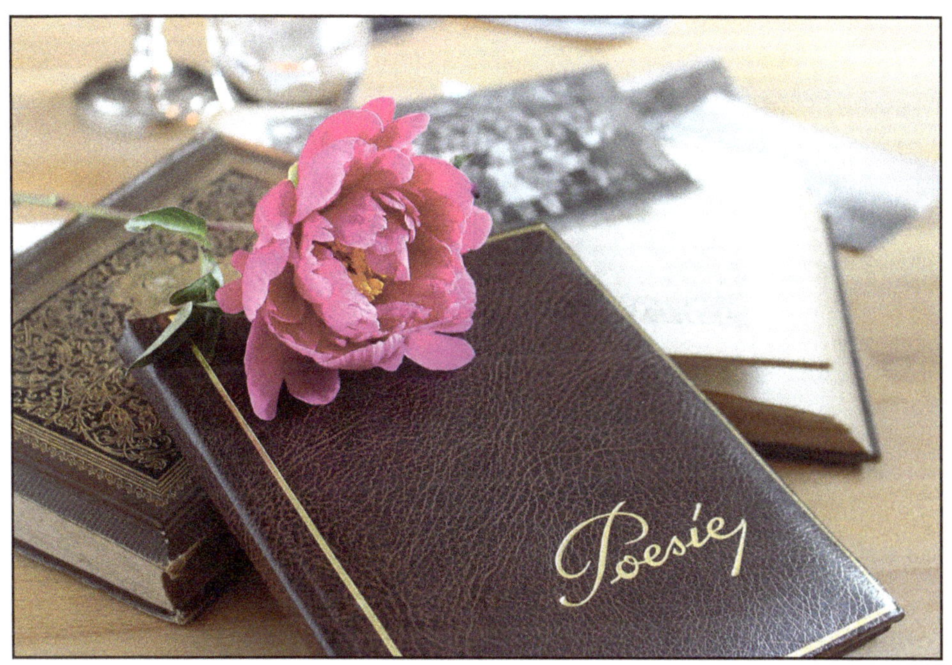

Manual Poetry Tools

My Orphan Children

There are some of my children
Who can't stand the light of day
It's not for what they are
But rather for what they say

It's not that they're not true
It's not that they're not real
It's not that they won't do
They show too much of how I feel

And sometimes they include
A friend of mine held close
And of my feelings for this friend
They contain a double dose

Sometimes they contain facts
Of which I am truly ashamed
Sometimes they contain feelings
Which remain as yet untamed

Sometimes a single quatrain
Says something hard to explain
And the secret it does contain
Is a thing propriety can't sustain

So these children of mine stay hidden
I don't let them out into the light
I make them keep their own counsel
Even though doing so might not be right

There may come a day in the future
When I feel these rhymes no longer offend
And these secret children of mine now hidden
Can come out in the open in the end

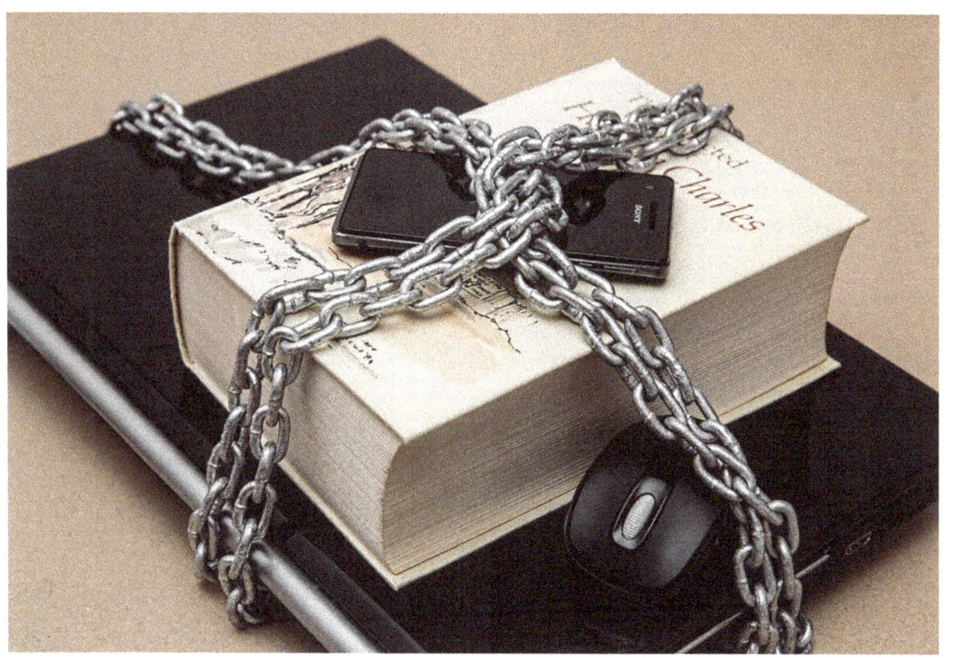

Reserved For The Future

Listening to Self Talk

When it comes to conversation
There's one kind that's highly prized
That's valued for it's erudition
Even when logic is capsized

It is short on argumentation
And so is often enjoyed
Can be of short duration
Thus it often is employed

Seldom gets hung up on semantics
And it requires but little proof
It always allows for verbal antics
Can withstand a strong reproof

Requires a quorum of but one
And so is easily conducted
Is often over before it's begun
No expert's fee deducted

There's no need for amplification
The voice is usually self contained
No need for writing or dictation
Disagreement is usually restrained

There is usually no noted distraction
Unless there are multiple personalities
In which cases there may be a reaction
Requiring the law and legal formalities

But generally there's an attempt
To arrive at a satisfactory conclusion
Without generating self contempt
Or laboring under a delusion

There's always an attempt at reconciliation
Of the facts and surrounding situation
An assessment of the issue's causation
An attempt to understand its formation

While there are occasionally questions
There are seldom seen protestations
Few requests are made for explanations
Little thought is given to the implications

The main resource is quiet reflection
Seldom needed is deft deflection
Based entirely on personal perception
The product is basic self protection

Seldom sought is veracity
No the truth is not highly prized
The output can be mendacity
Self service is thinly disguised

Now I don't mean to imply
That all self talk is self serving
The truth does not always die
Sometimes self talk is deserving

But at the very heart of the matter
That is, when all is said and done
Self talk is sometimes idle chatter
Yet it seems the verbal war is won

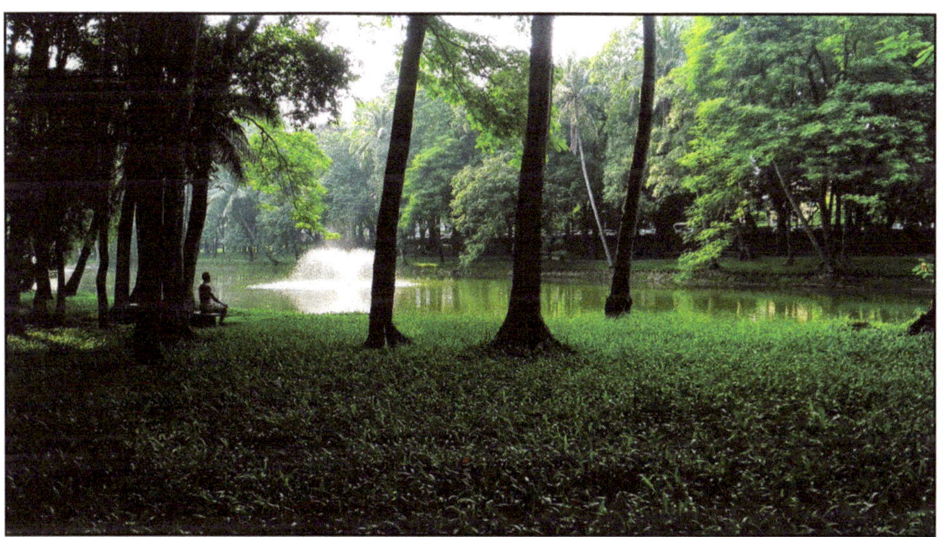

Self Talk-Meditation

Simply Haiku

Just five syllables
Followed by just seven more
Presto! A Haiku

Haiku Number Two

Golden Daffodil
Turned its trumpet toward the sun
Haiku number two

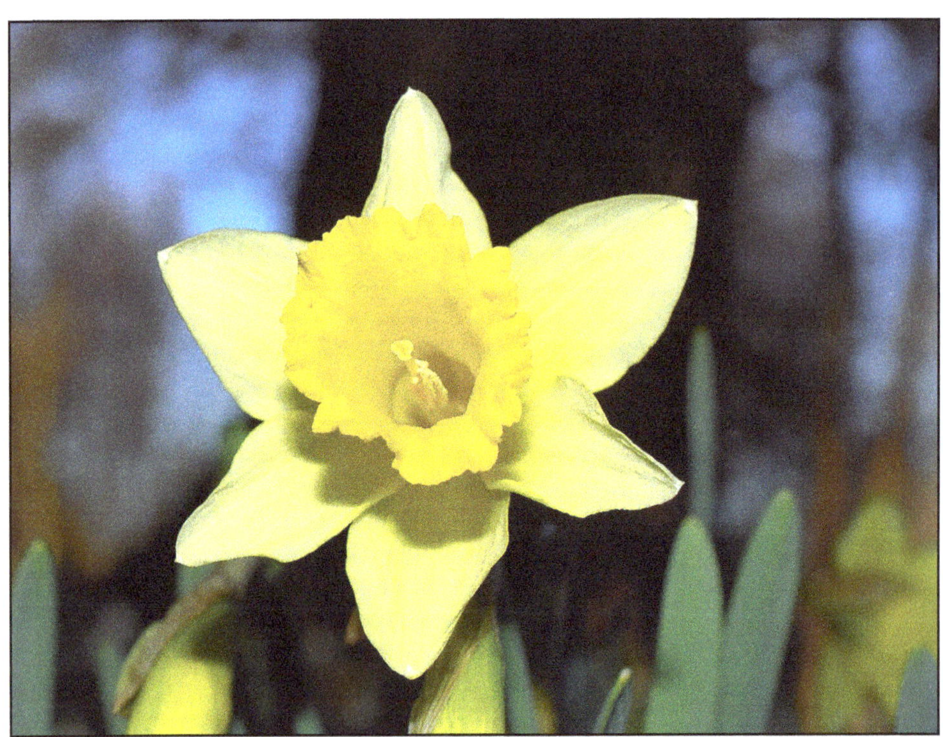

Daffodil

Ode to the Onomatopoeia

Inspiration by Susan Kirby

A friend of mine sounded me out
About writing an onomatopoeia poem
Such a work, I said, would be a flop
So I'll write one just to show 'em

I will collect all the examples I find
And store them away for later use
With a whistle and a whimper I'll secure 'em
So the meows and moos don't get loose

Tintinnabulation is a word I would choose
Just 'cause Poe found it so incredibly saucy
I'd put it in a pail of water, kerplop
Just to try to keep it good and glossy

The water so cold would splash up
And it would catch me all unaware
I, in turn, would sneeze all achoo
Keep the word there should a sound flair

I'd travel on in search of more words
Sneak an onomatopoeia here and there
I'd slap them in my bucket with a huff
Gargle, giggle, and gobble would be there

Then I'd search for some animal sounds
I'd scarf up arf, bark, cackle, caw, and coo
I'd continue to fill my bucket of words
I'd choose bleat, cheep, chirp, and hiss too

And then to provide some melody to the mix
I'd wrestle in chime, clang, oompah, and toot
I'd also gather ding-a-ling, twang, and gong
And beep, bloop, bong, buzz, and blare to boot

And now we need to add some action to the pail
So I'll search for blip, blow, boing and bounce
I'd choose chug, crack, and creak along with drizzle
Rattle, rumble, and squirt lend more sound to the ounce

And now that I've gathered all these sounds
Dare I ask you what does it matter?
For I can't hear myself think
Above all of this clatter

So I'll use this pail to some avail
To water the verbal vegetation
For this bucket of words lends life
To the written word and all its declarations

From the sounds of it
I've completed my quest
Even if I have not
I have done my level best

Now I'll sit here in silence
And wait for the reaction
We'll see if anyone claps
Or shows signs of satisfaction

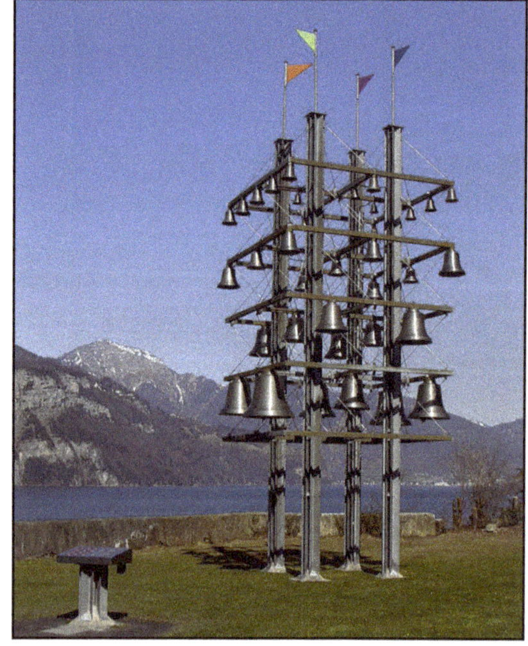

*The Sound Bells Make
When They Ring*

Imagination

Imagine if you will
I certainly do
I Consider things that aren't
Like dinosaurs at the zoo

Imagine wearing white
After Labor Day
A white organza suit
No matter what they say

What of a flock of birds
All without wings?
You can imagine this
Among many other things

Imagine an elephant
Getting himself a drink
With each of his two trunks
Should this cause one to blink?

Pay attention to an oak
Bearing pink pineapples
Wouldn't they yield a drink
More desirable than apples?

How about a stapler
That never runs out of staples
An endless supply of wire
No need to move it from the table

And what of a big black bear
With a glowing golden furry coat?
Would the other bears object
If this odd bear were to gloat?

Imagination yields all sorts
Of rare and odd manifestations
Grist and meal enough
To rock all of our foundations

What of an ear of corn
Without its silky tassel
Could you accept it
Without a harried hassle?

Imagination makes sometimes
For strange bedfellows
Like the tasteless chunks
Of metallic marshmallows

Imagine a leafless book
If you have a mind
Would you give it a second look?
Could you read it if you're blind?

And what of a catcher's mitt
Made to look just like an oven's
The work of a wicked witch
And others from her coven

Consider how common words
Contribute to imagination
What if a potato did have eyes
Would that yield a visual sensation?

I hesitate to suggest this
But what of a flywheel
Can you imagine its function
If all the flies were real?

What if a bottled up harbor
Were bottled up with bottles?
Could the sailor escape its grip
By laying on the throttle?

Can you even imagine
A blanket of snow?
Much easier than shoveling
You'd fold it back you know

And what if pies
Were really made of mud
Some would get a big surprise
Others would get a dud

Imagine being able
To see into the dark
You could walk at midnight
Tan in the moon glow on a lark

You could always
Bring friends back from the dead
Then there would be
No funerals to dread

With imagination
There simply are no rules
Anything that you can think of
Fantasy and invention are your tools

Conjure up an animal
Of any strange description
You could make yourself a pet
Of your mind's favorite depiction

Oh, imagination's function
When you first employ it
Has reality on the run
Now you can enjoy it

I really could go on
From here until forever
Forsaking what we know
And conforming to convention never

I refuse to rely
On the written rules
Rather than comply
I'll use imagination and fancy for my tools

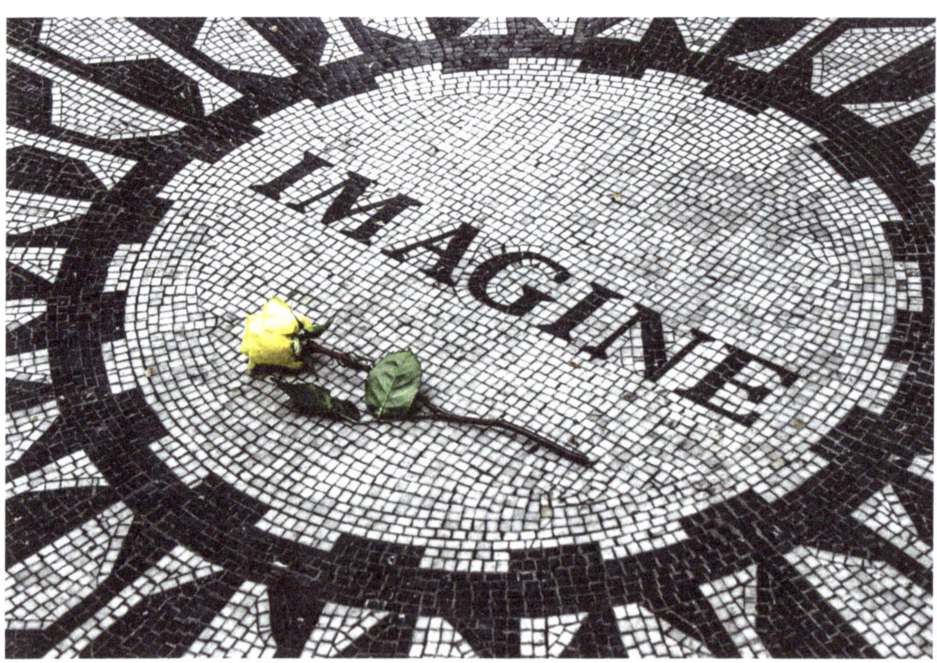

Plato Poetry Pandering

Plato wasn't particularly pro poetry
Fact is, he didn't even like it
Felt it didn't reflect true reality
Rather than read, he would spike it

So I thought I would undertake the impossible
And try to write a poem Plato palatable
I will try to address his concern of the incognoscible*
While plying philosophical waters navigable

A case of controlled Platonic perception
You see, that is what here I'm aiming for
Avoidance of false facts and outright deception
Truth and objective reality is all I'll explore

I will avoid flowery descriptions
And neural musings of any kind
Won't focus on mere mental depictions
Those things conjured up in my mind

Fact is I don't know where I'm going
I find myself in a quite serious bind
There's more I don't know than I'm knowing
I'm proceeding as though I were blind

A further fact is, I don't understand his objection
Unless he just liked to argue the metaphysical
To the sights and sounds which influenced perception
That in turn inspired the poetic works typical

In an effort to remain with this task and not stray
I certainly shall remain, in the main, engaged
Yes, with this work I remain committed to stay
And in the end will have a full blown effort waged

Plato, it seems, consistently objected on the basis
Of three academic features in a state of stasis
Education, philosophy, and finally morality
Arguing for each alone, and all in totality

The first point of objection was education
Poetry was not a haven of good habit cultivation
Homer's epics were full of cunning, cruelty, and lust
Trying to teach good clean living from them is a bust

And then there was the philosophical argument
If you don't grasp this point there will be no punishment
Philosophy deals with the ultimate reality – the truth
Poetry, though, was truth twice removed and presented to youth

Art to Plato is simply an illusion
A structured attempt at delusion
This is his theory of mimesis**
The truth to him is more precious

And finally we come to morality in its season
The higher principles of man revolve around reason
Poetry, though, appeals to impulses and emotions
According to Plato there's less value to these notions

In his famous profound allegory
Plato tells us another story
Those who would not be a slave
Have to emerge from the cave

For the shadows projected on the wall
Are not what's true but mimesis all
And the shadows are like poetic art
Make it hard to tell truth and delusion apart

And thus he explains succinctly the interference
Of poet and philosopher, their products' appearance
While the poet describes the shadows on the wall
The philosopher leaves the cave and explains it all

Despite my promise to address his concern with the incognoscible
I have proven myself incapable of mastering what is impossible
For it seems I, at length, am forced to finally admit
Plato's smarter than me, by a hair, to that I commit

It was presumptuous to contemplate
That I could write a Plato Poem
But I hope you can commiserate
With me if you just know him

**incapable of being perceived or known*
***representation or imitation of the real world in art and literature.*

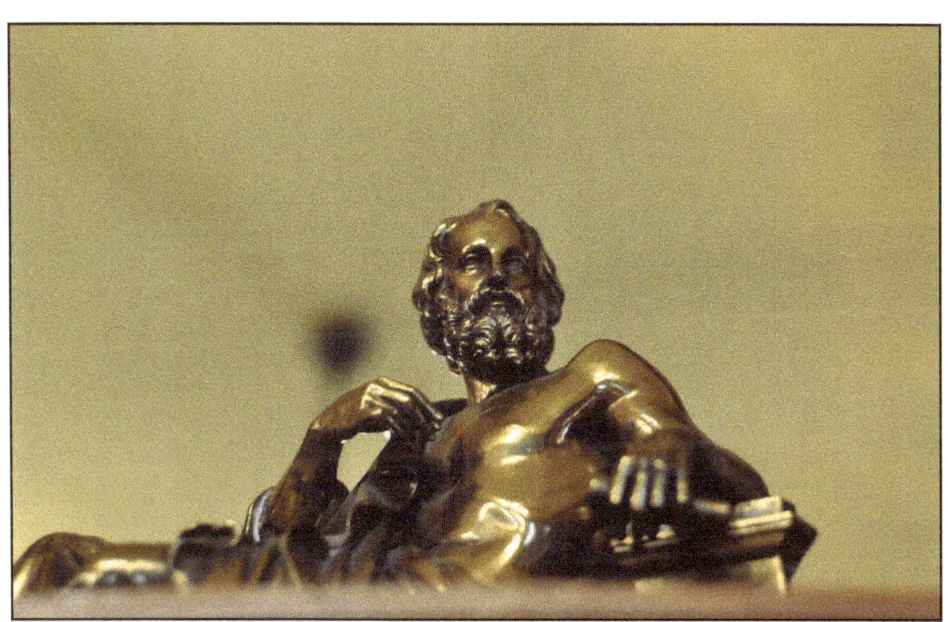

Plato

What Do You Know - Portmanteau

It occurs to me that you can look at portmanteau
In one of two very different ways
As a suitcase or the means of forming new words
Like taxicab from taximeter and cabriolet

Words I find are much more fun
Than some old leather suitcases
So let's look at some common words
And see just what their source is

It's fun to find fairly fancy examples, too
Of words that are portmanteaux
Like melatonin from melanin and serotonin
Good for sleep we'd rather not forgo

And who doesn't enjoy a good cyborg
Featured in many a child's comic book
A joining of cybernetic and organism
Yet we've accepted it without a second look

Consider a common word like TaeBo
Do you even know where the word comes from?
It's a portmanteau from Taekwondo and boxing
If you didn't know, no reason you should feel glum

A more exotic word is cermet
And where do you think this one comes from?
It also is a portmanteau of ceramic and metal
To the beauty of this method you may yet succumb

Here's another compounded word
It's a simple portmanteau
Made from carbon and corundum
Carborundum is the word you know

Next up is a very common word
It's plain old motorcade
It may surprise you how it's made
Comes from motor and cavalcade

Genome is a popular word
And it, of course, is a portmanteau
It comes from gene and chromosome
Knowing this may cause some braggadocio

You've no doubt had pointed out, the contrail of a jet
But did you know that that portmanteau
Was made up of condensation and trail?
That's something else that you now know

We've all heard that our mood is affected by endorphins
But you may be surprised to learn of its verbal source
Which is listed as endogenous and morphine
And you guessed it, it's a portmanteau of course

In an attempt to rid one's face of wrinkles
Many try regular injections of Botox
The word comes from botulism and toxin
An odd practice since we usually want to detox

Consider jazzercise if you will
Made up, of course, of jazz and exercise
Shows portmanteau need not be static
Just that two words it must comprise

Another example of portmanteau is surfactant
I didn't know until I looked it up by chance
I didn't recognize surface and active agent
It just wasn't obvious at first glance

Some portmanteaux are obscure
Take for instance the word snuba
I had never heard it before
It is made from snorkel and scuba

Other words are very common
Motocross comes to mind
Motor and cross country
These two are combined

I think that by now the point is made
So, if you're game, let's find a way out of here
What do you say we try parasailing
From parachute and sailing, off we go without fear

Definition of portmanteau
1: a large suitcase
2: a word blending the sounds and combining the meanings of two others

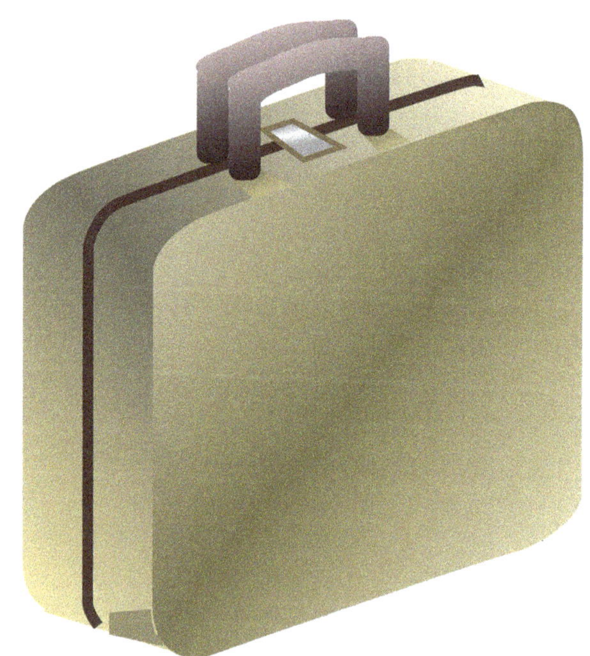

A Portmanteau
of Portmanteauz

In Search of Inspiration (Pastor Bob)

I am searching for a topic
But seem artistically myopic
No other author would I rob
So I settled on plain old Bob

Bob happens to be a friend of mine
It seems I see him all the time
Hear he is well versed in scripture
That he paints a pretty verbal picture

Often tease him that he's evil
That his theories are Medieval
He brings the worst out in me
With his "come on" proclivity

I tease him about his shoes
There's so little left to lose
I tease him about most things
Attached there are no strings

I truly enjoy our conversations
Despite cerebral calculations
It's fun to posture and match wits
Though we can give each other fits

Bob, it is said, is a man of the cloth
I do my best to lead him away from sloth
I, in fact, try to help him avoid all vices
Safer than leaving him to his own devices

Sometimes Bob gets somewhat confused
And takes a notion that I'm to be abused
While I know him to be contentious
I doubt the claims that he's licentious

There's a fine line 'twixt the irreverent and factual
With Bob I always try to present what is actual
That, you see, is what I have tried to do here
To the truth I have tried my best to come near

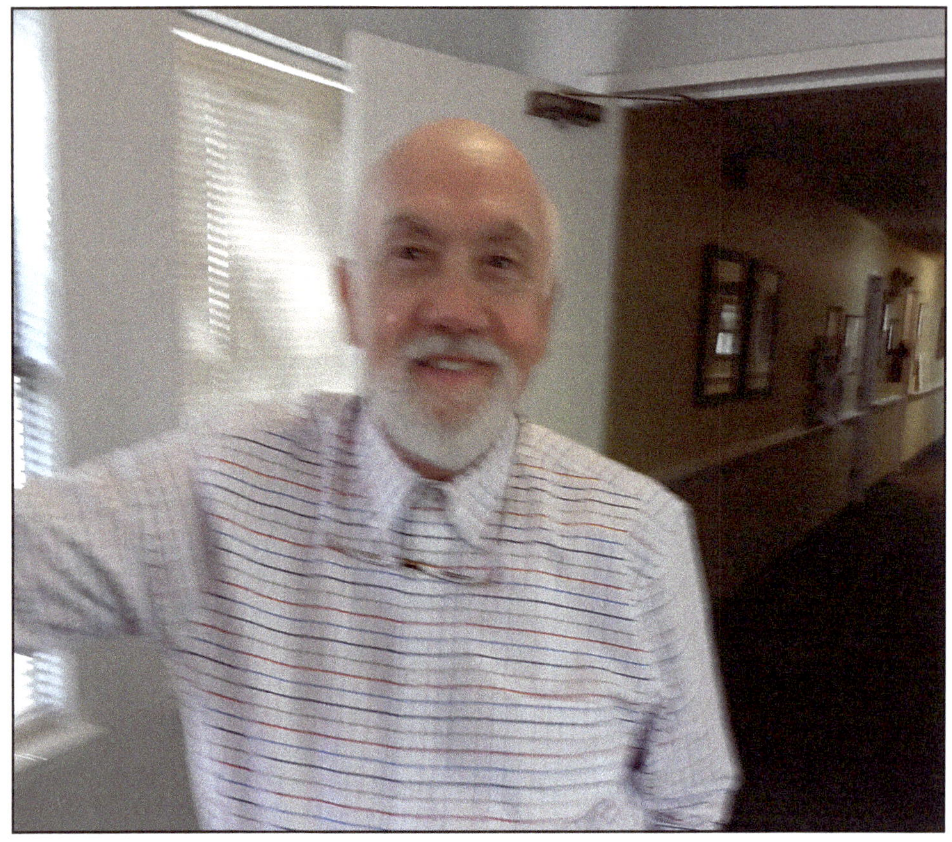

Pastor Bob Hopkins

CHAPTER SIX
The Nurses

Just a Few Simple Tributes

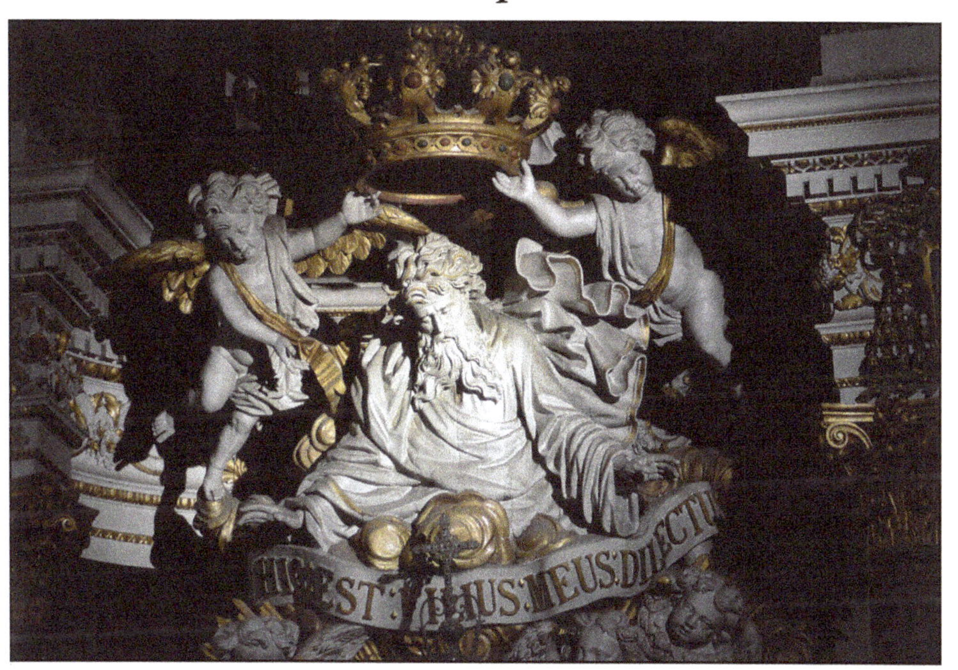

A Choir of Angels

A New Nurse (Emily)

A new nurse came on the scene today
And we all pray that she will stay
She's quick witted and efficient
In no way is she deficient

Long blonde hair and a pleasant smile
We all hope she'll last awhile
Beautiful and very friendly
She improves our moods immensely

Tall and thin and quite wasp waisted
No way she can be overrated
She, it seems, is always cheerful
When giving shots she's very skillful

She reminds one of Nightingale
Rated on a sliding scale
She comes in at, or near, the top
My praise for her no one can stop

And so as she gets off the mark
And on this job does embark
We wish her well quite completely
Careful to praise her most discreetly

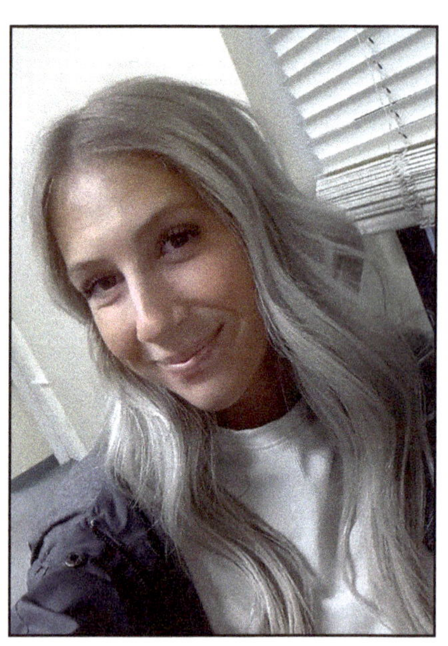

Emily McFarland

DRK
(Rene)

Diana Renee Kilgore is her full name
And compassionate nursing is her game
She was born in Dunlap, one of four
Of her it can be said, "she cares a little more"

Don't let her small size fool you
Her smile is going to rule you
She has an over sized heart
You'll notice that from the start

She is certainly very proficient
Her methods are most efficient
She pays attention to all the details
Her concern for the best never fails

She was the first person I met when I came here
I knew then that life would not be the same here
She was kind and took time to pay attention
She performed her work without pretension

Everyone knows she loves June, her standard poodle
When she's with her, attempts at distraction are futile
While any attempt to refute it would be rash
We all know she still loves her old friend, Cash*

When she isn't tending to chores
Rene enjoys spending time out of doors
It seems that she almost always is busy
The pace she keeps would make you dizzy

She almost always wears her hair up
Her temper I've never seen flare up
She has a kind and gentle disposition
She's a great adjunct to a physician

I recently damaged my pill minder
Renee could not have been kinder
She emptied it and loaded a new one
She's an angel if ever I knew one

Once when I was walking too much
With my Psych Nurse Practitioner she got in touch
She needn't have bothered, I had no complaint
She got involved simply because she is a saint

I said it before, you know she's kind
If you can't see that you're surely blind
That she cares you should have no doubt
It's her basic nature I'm talking about

* *Cash is a male standard poodle that once lived with Rene and June*

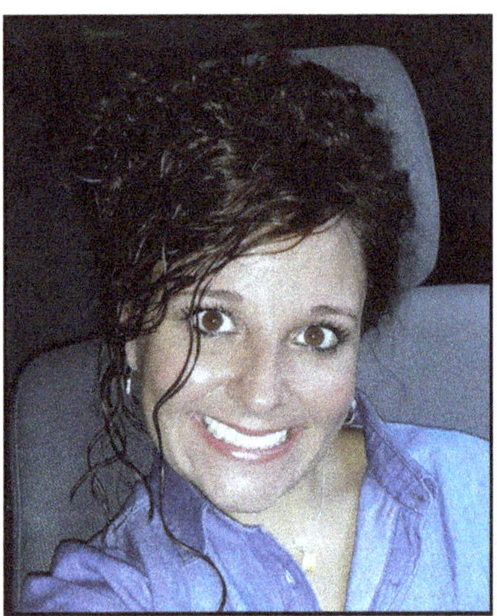

Rene Kilgore

Starlight Star Bright (Star)

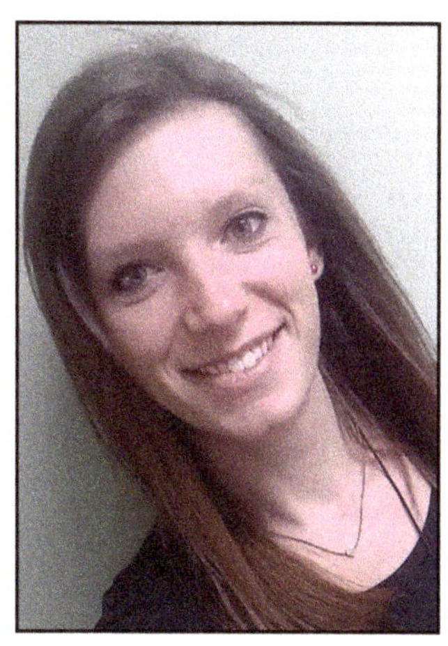

Starlana Camp

Star burst on our scene unexpectedly
She stole our hearts quite effectively
It didn't hurt at all that she was beautiful
That she was right for the job was indisputable

She has a very delightful sense of humor
That she could master any task was the rumor
She did far more than just hand out pills
Her kind nature tended to cure many ills

Many days her "Good Mornings" lifted my spirits
Especially when my blues had reached their limits
She could do more with one of her simple smiles
The whole host of geriatric inmates she beguiles

She was nothing less than a bright supernova
She had the athleticism of Martina Navratilova
Many of us wished we'd seen her play softball
As she does in her work, she must have given it her all

Her attention to detail was, to say the least, stellar
This fact was appreciated by each facility dweller
She never promised to do a thing and then failed
Her honesty and perseverance were both hailed

To know her made you want to study astrophysics
She made you want to master all the specifics
Of a science that deals strictly with heavenly bodies
And of all the space that that science embodies

For in the end, you see, she left us*
There's simply nothing to discuss
Except how to fill the black holes
She left in our hearts and our souls

** Star returned on a PRN basis*

CHAPTER SEVEN
Dreams

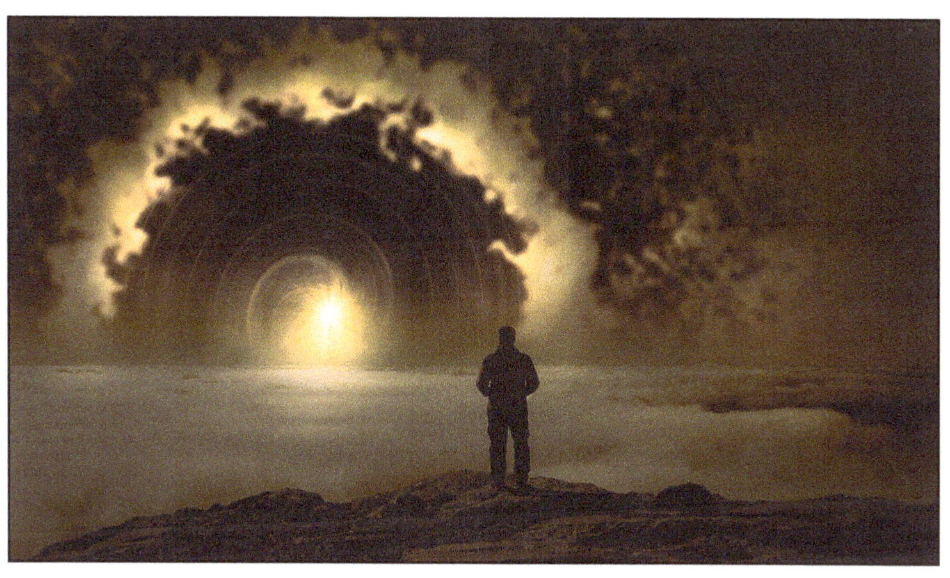

How I Dream Or How It Seems

The Detour

I had a strange dream last night
I didn't understand it quite
It was rooted in my old school days
Surrounded in fog, enveloped in haze

It started with a penalty assessed
That in the end was not addressed
It centered first on my school library
Which used to be my sanctuary

I had been assigned a fine
For not returning a book in time
I know it seems a simple matter
But my self esteem it didn't flatter

I began the day headed to class
But soon found myself in a morass
It seems, you see, I lost my way
On my way to class that day

I found myself on a broad boulevard
Which appeared to me as a vast courtyard
Lining the street were rows of castles
Felt I'd become one of the vassals

The walls were all crenelated
The kings were all checkmated
The knights were all mounted
Their enemies surmounted

The walls of the castles were all of stone
The armor on the brave knights shone
The drawbridges were all drawn up tight
As if they had been set up for the knight

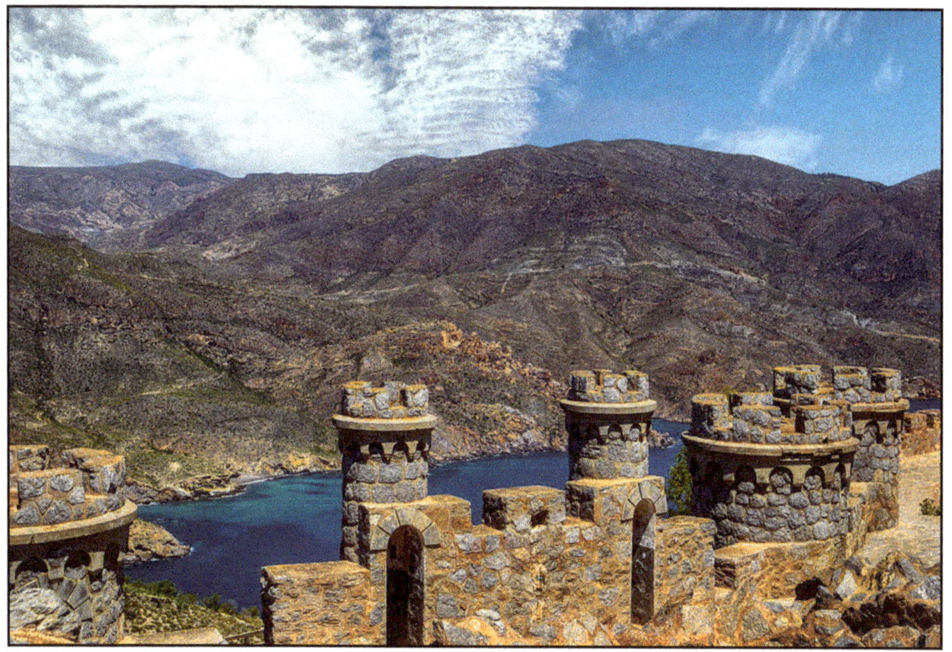

One of The Many Castles

I wandered among these unknown spaces
Until I came to familiar places
I headed off to school in haste
"Must make up for the time I waste"

When I left home that day
I was obsessed by the fine to pay
I hurried to the library, see
To pay the dues, the assessed fee

Due to my detour I was late
And wound up outside the gate
Only to find my fine erased
My reputation not defaced

Because I was late
The fine they'd negate
You'd have thought they'd be inclined
To increase the size of the fine

But there was something about
That detour that I took
That caused them to give
The thing a second look

Where had I been that had this effect
The negation of the fine they'd select
This side trip to a medieval kingdom
Helped in some way to pay my ransom

So what lesson should I divine
From this dream of mine so sublime
I wish someone could help me see
Just what this dream means for me

Joe Smith

The Hall of Many Doors

I walked down a hall last night
I was awake yet I was dreaming
Some of what I saw gave me a fright
I knew my muddled mind was scheming

Some of what I saw was benign
Some of what I saw was repulsive
Some things I saw I can't define
Some things made me convulsive

I'm well aware my mind plays tricks
And this episode could be delusion
Brain chemicals could be in the mix
Deprivation and addled brain in collusion

I started down the hall real slow
There were doors on either side
What was behind each I didn't know
And my curiosity I couldn't abide

So I knocked on each in turn
Hoping to gain admittance
Trying my best to slowly learn
Without paying a remittance

At my knock the first door yielded
Yes it swung open fairly wide
I stared wide eyed at what was wielded
By the specter that was inside

In his hand there was a log book
Leather bound and most official
At my request the specter let me look
The first thing I saw was my initials

The book appeared to be a record
Of all the mistakes I'd ever made
Not one it seemed had been ignored
Not even those for which I'd paid

I decided it best to avoid confusion
So I'd label this door "Regrets"
For I had come to the conclusion
That these were things I'd never forget

I begged the specter's gracious pardon
And then proceeded on down the hall
I dressed up in my spirit most Spartan
Needed for the next door, the most painful of all

I approached the next door with trepidation
Deathly afraid of what I might there find
This turned out to be a somewhat different situation
One that would leave me caught in a bind

As this door slowly swung open
I felt a shiver run up my spine
Inside were feelings unspoken
About loves lost over time

The specter in charge of these memories
Was a heartless and cruel master
She sought to cement the treacheries
Involved in my most personal disasters

She showed me films of girls and women
That had been more than close in the past
Who had in the end made the decision
That the love we had wouldn't last

Though this was the most painful door
It was in fact somewhat bittersweet
Though these subjects I came to adore
I never came to the point of loss complete

I still hold visions of them in my heart
Even though that may seem strange
They simply always will be a part
Of the "Loves Lost" lonely exchange

As I moved slowly but surely down the hall
I stopped and wondered what I'd find next
I thought "these doors are but holes in the wall"
I surely shouldn't let my mind be vexed

Still the specters that inhabited the rooms
Had a way of grabbing my attention
Spreading as they did immortal gloom
And filling my mind with apprehension

Feeling fearful, fretful, and lost
I felt my way down the corridor
Hoping to find peace at any cost
Might it be found at the next door?

Knocking softly at the next portal
I held my heart high in my throat
I was feeling oh so mortal
My intuition I wouldn't demote

The specter that answered this door
Was more casual than all the rest
He held a ball, bat, slingshot and more
Of all the specters I liked him best

It was apparent he had come to show me
What it apparently was like to be a child
And at first it seemed he didn't know me
But after a short while he went wild

He started off by duplicating
Mistakes I'd made as a youth
There were fistfights and adjudicating
There were arguments over the truth

There were trips made to the family swimming pool
There were excursions to parks both far and wide
All the time attempts were made at the Golden Rule
"Childhood Memories" was the name on which I would decide

"Regrets", "Love's Lost", and "Childhood Memories"
I recognized these addresses, while accurate, overlapped
But I also recognized that there were likely other reveries
Which up until this time had surely not been mapped

In search of these other reveries
I finally set about to find
Surely among all these memories
I'd find or lose my mind

I slowed my hall advancement
To no more than a crawl
I had experienced some enchantment
At that last childish port of call

I earlier indicated that "Loves Lost"
Was the most painful door of them all
But next there came a door at high cost
A door that would cause my flesh to crawl

The specter that answered my truly timid but timely knock
Was a cretaceous creature possessed of two tremendous heads
Note that this door unlike the others was guarded by a lock
Which made a good deal of sense since he could tear a man to shreds

The specter moved steadily but slow
With each head bobbing side to side
It was hard to tell which way he would go
Each step he took his path he belied

In his left hand he held a sharp dagger
A club covered with spikes in his right
When he tried to walk he would stagger
From his four eyes there shone a bright light

Both of his hands were copiously covered in blood
He smelled of sulfur, gangrene, and burnt flesh
There were scars on his arms which were covered in crud
Nothing about this cadaverous creature was fresh

Hung on the wall were barbed whips and chains
In the furthest corner of the room was a rack
Everything about this creature spelled pain
There were two rows of spikes on his back

I had obviously entered the room of my "Fears"
As soon as I entered I just wanted out
Just looking at the creature brought me to tears
I wasn't sure what this scene was about

Wisely, I thought, I quickly retreated
Into the dank, dingy, dimly lit hall
This scene I hoped wouldn't be repeated
For I now thought it worst of them all

I had begun to feel the painful toll
Of my various special spectral visits
I suddenly felt much less than whole
A fragmented feeling these visits elicit

I thought of the dated popular rhyme
"Come into my parlor said the spider to the fly"
Though I felt I was running out of time
I thought the fly could conquer the spider by and by

So I made up my mind to try
Just one more mysterious entry
Into the parlor like the fabulous fly
And visit with another sentry

Again the door yielded at my knock
And swung slowly silently open
The boat I was careful not to rock
No rules up to now I had broken

The specter that inhabited this room
Was larger than any contemporary
There was about him a feeling of doom
Of all the specters, of him I was most wary

I had the response of fight or flight
I didn't think he was there just to talk
I knew something wasn't quite right
I felt I should turn and quickly walk

I perceived an unfriendly or angry air
As I gazed quickly about the room
There was a definite presence there
As I mentioned, a sensation of doom

In the dim light I could barely make out
A congregation of my former adversaries
I knew immediately what they were about
They caused the constriction of my capillaries

For I quickly recognized
These as my sworn opponents
And just as soon I realized
I couldn't stay another moment

I know not why they congregated there
But I was sure it wasn't me admiration
I knew for sure I shouldn't stay where
A bellicose event could be given causation

Once again I retreated into the hall
In search of self preservation
I wasn't about to take the fall
And cause my self cessation

About this time I got a clear clue
I wasn't welcome in this hall at all
If anything my departure was due
If only my demise to forestal

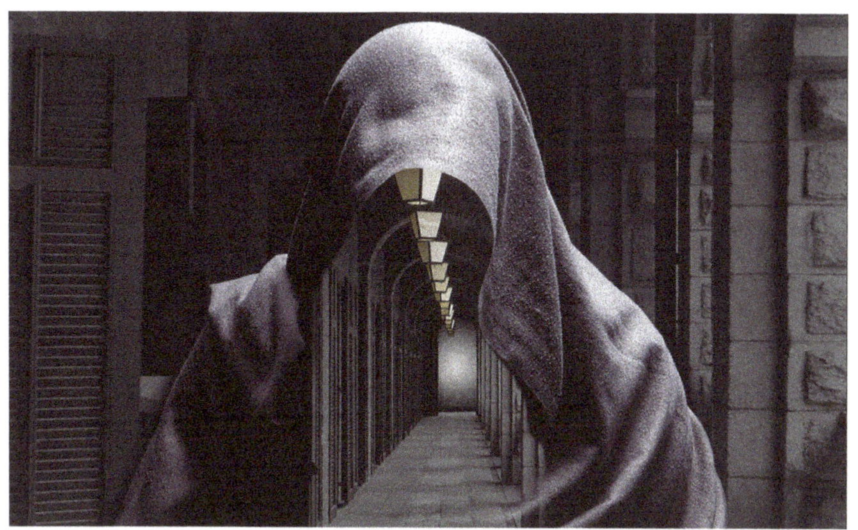

The Hall of Many Doors

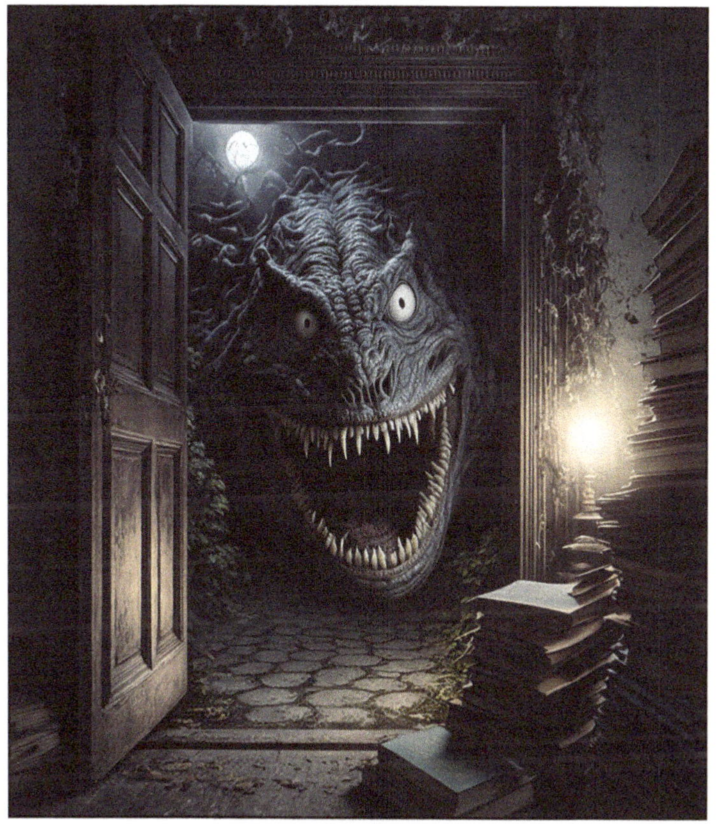

One of the Monster's Two Heads

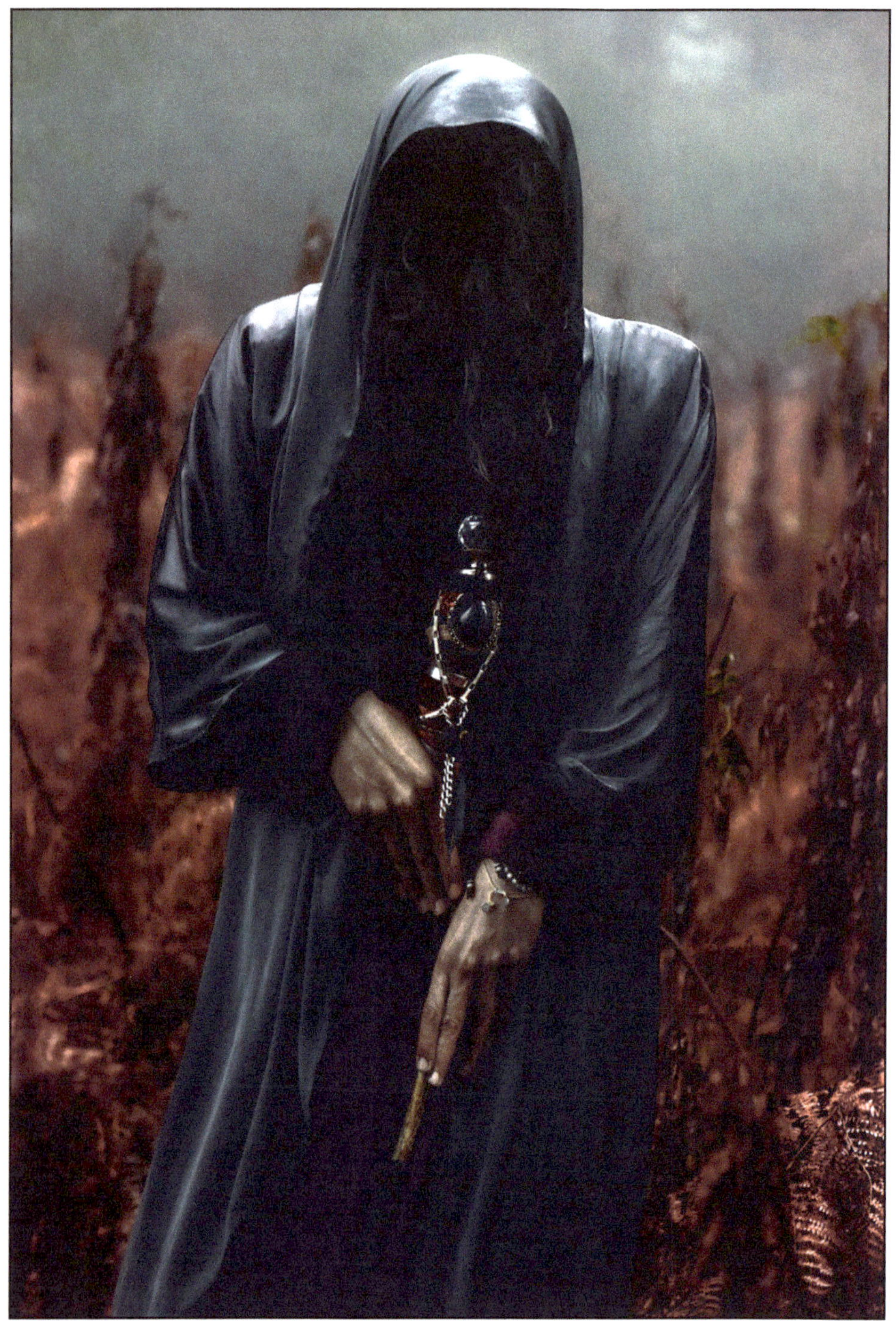

A Specter From the Hall of Many Doors

CHAPTER EIGHT
Miscellaneous

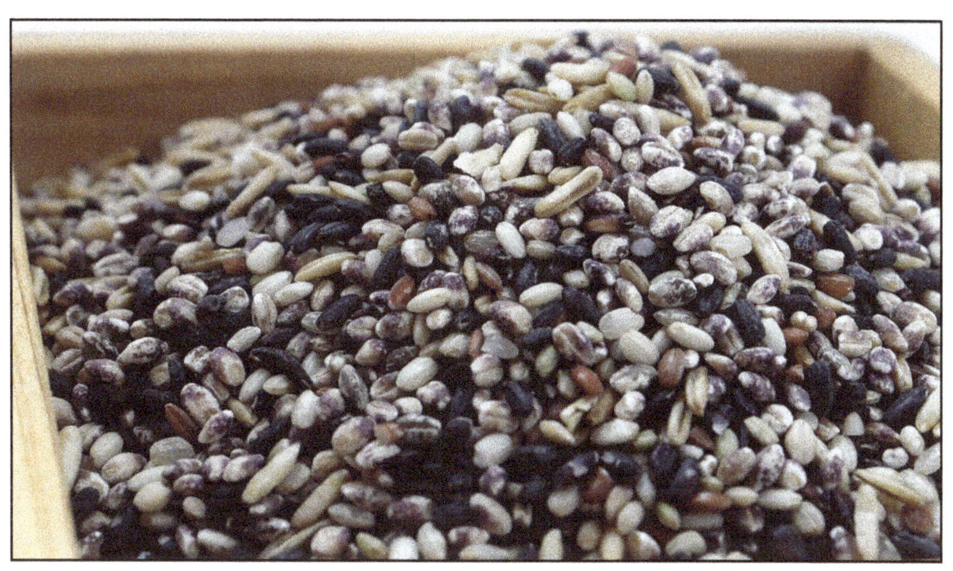

A Healthy Mix

Up On Two Wheels

This is a poem about a bicycle
A most basic form of transportation
It won't be easy to write this one
It can't stand on its own as inspiration

When I was but a wee small lad
My life's plan in incubation
I would travel far and wide
To relieve life's irritation

The bike always provided me
With a means of safe escape
I traveled many a carefree mile
To escape the odd tight scrape

The bike gave me a sense of freedom
When simply nothing else could
I'd pedal from problems aimlessly
Despite whether or not I should

The bicycle took me out of the neighborhood
And gave me a highly prized sense of elation
It gave me a highly prized sense of freedom too
More than any other form of transportation

I traveled far and wide 'cross the city
And visited all of the major parks
I roamed distant neighborhoods
Often visited friends of mine on larks

Many was the day when I rose before the rest
And pedaled up and down the street
And then I, it seems, tried my level best
The early onset of the blues to beat

My bike back then was my friend
It kept my life, you see, in balance
And now I know that in the end
It prevented emotional imbalance

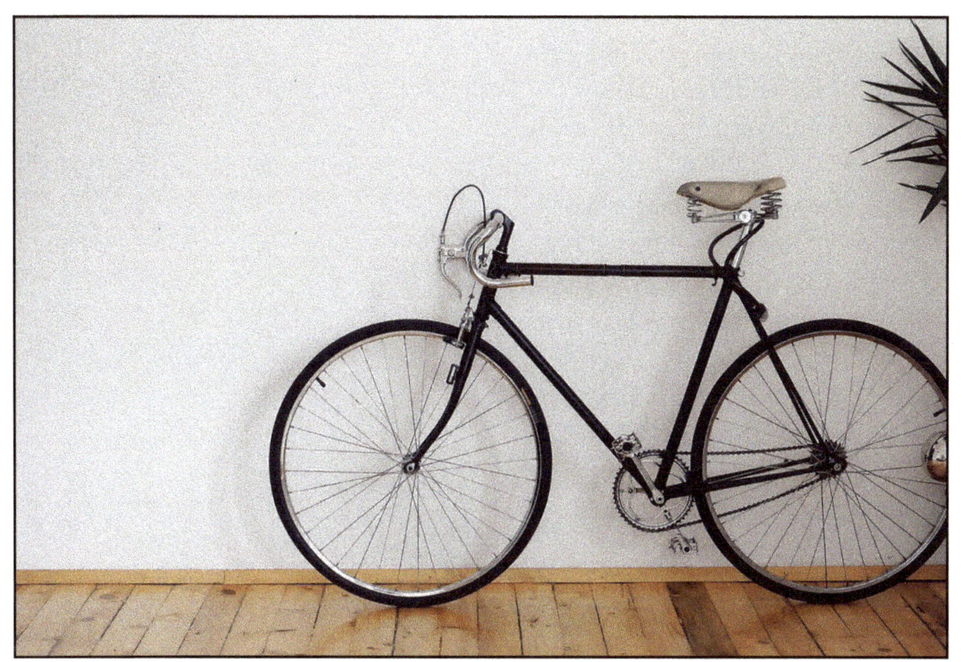

A Matter of Balance

Treasure Chest or Pandora's Box

I have a box upon my shelf
It's been there fifty years
It contains something of myself
My youthful hopes and fears

In the box there are some letters
Written by a sixteen year old girl
About a love with no fetters
About giving communal life a whirl

I remember some word for word
So deeply they had impressed me
Of some I wish I had never heard
Those in turn, it seems, now depress me

Now I find myself debating
Should I open the box and see
If there are any clues relating
To why our love ceased to be

Or will I be truly uplifted
By the sentiments that there I find
From the thoughts that are there to be sifted
Will I find all of them kind

Will the letters contain in them clues
As to why we, in the end, didn't make it
It's more than a matter of who we choose
I'm not sure now I can take it

There was a certain degree of commitment
In her writing to me every day
For my part I wrote daily also
Though I sometimes had little to say

Before taking a chance on inspection
Of these missives of ancient device
I wonder if she has a collection
Of my letters to her to suffice

You see we both wrote daily
For the months I was away at school
To keep in close touch mainly
Daily contact was the rule

I never felt hard pressed to write them
I was happy to do it in fact
True, not all of the letters were gems
But emotion made up for what the words lacked

I'll point out here I was just eighteen
At the time this correspondence transpired
In just two years we would be married
And the letter exchange retired

I left the school of my choice to return home
So that we could be together again
The catalog of my new school I did comb
For classes near where I had been

I changed majors a few times
Uncertain of what I should do
But as sure as my ardor did climb
My involvement in school did too

But all of that is just history
To explain the situation we were in
Now comes the time to face the mystery
Of the aging of the letters in the bin

Remember these letters document
The beginning of our life together
We considered them the cement
That would hold us together forever

So now I think I will unlock
Treasure chest or Pandora's box
My memories I will thus unblock
After fifty years I've run out the clock

So I'll pause now in writing this piece
And review some of the letters
To see if my mood does increase
Or if it doesn't get any better
-
-
--
My review of the correspondence is now complete
Although I only reviewed a few of the posts
In dedication and emotion they were replete
But inhabited by portents and ghosts

Promises of undying affection
Filled each and every page
No hint of the later defection
Of discontent and unbridled rage

I had to limit my meddlesome intake
Of the words I finally found there
I had to cease review for my own sake
For I found that I still harbored care

Despite my every effort
To remain aloof and detached
I found myself without comfort
As I reviewed each and every dispatch

I found I had to take the opportunity
To dry my eyes each and every time
I read of promised unity
Separation it seemed was a crime

There were records of brief excursions
When our souls surely would blend
Sum and substance of incursions
That we hoped would never end

There was an incident recorded
In which there was a break
An incident so sordid
It paused our daily give and take

I don't recall the story
Or any of its facts
It seems there was no glory
In the play or in its acts

In a letter she accepts responsibility
For the interrupted correspondence
She allows for no possibility
That I caused her deep despondence

Instead she accepts the blame
For having treated me unkind
It brought out in me a sense of shame
To think I was ever so blind

As to let her assume the blame
For something of this kind
It really is a crying shame
I must have been in a bind

But then again I have no record
Of how I might have responded
Was I in complete accord
What had I corresponded?

What else could be contained in here
That I had forgotten about?
This could be Pandora's box I fear
What monsters was I letting out?

But in truth there were some treasures
Contained within this chest
To be released in full measures
But are surely left alone best

Again, I wonder if she has a box
A box of memories like mine
I wonder if she picks the locks
And lets our true past shine

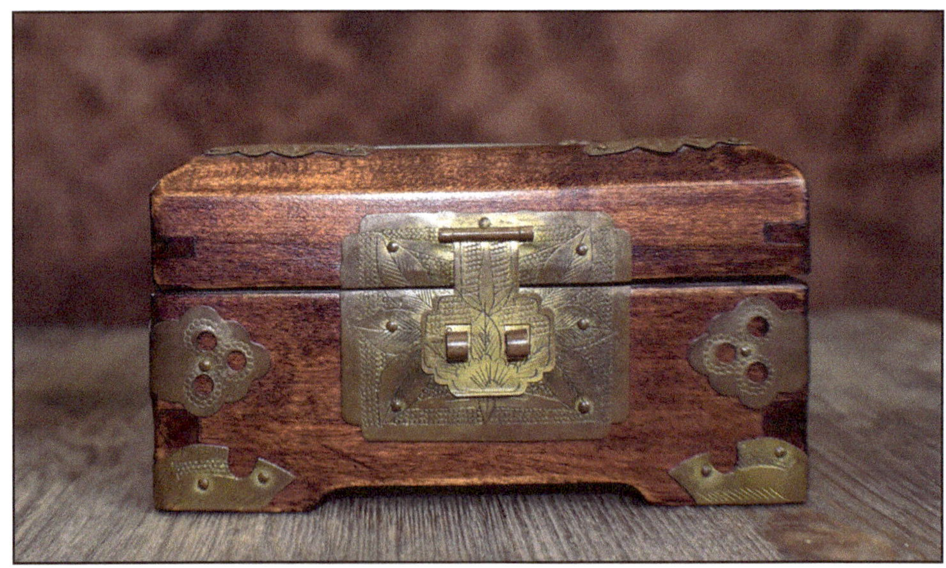

Pandora's Box?

"Does Anybody Really Know What Time It Is"

Inspired by Phyllis Baker

It seems we can't always agree
On just just what time it should be
It seems this AM it was 2 o'clock
And at the same time 3, a shock

It's something called DST
That leads this mystery to be
Yes it seems that Daylight Savings
Leads us to these contradictory cravings

And then, of course, there's all those time zones
Which cause more confusion, I make no bones
Eastern, Central, Mountain, and then Pacific
Make time hard to know unless you're specific

And in the Fall we change to Standard Time
Which causes the level of confusion to climb
At 2 in the morning it's suddenly 1 AM
True time is suddenly in question again

So knowing the true time is a question of when and where
The uncertainty of the situation is almost too much to bear
When someone asks you the time you surely best beware
For there are time and space features of which you must be aware

What does this all mean to watch and to clock
With which the great secret of time we hope to unlock?
There is always a question, too, of accuracy
The atomic clock in Boulder keeps track miraculously

We brag on our timepieces now and then
The British like to point to their Big Ben
There are those who value their Rolex
And some who brag of their Timex no less

There are other ways that we keep track of time
Some are just plain practical, others sublime
For instance we do use the calendar some
To keep track of days, weeks, and birthdays to come

But even the calendar is subject to interpretation
With six major types used, depending on the nation
Gregorian, Jewish, Islamic, Indian, Chinese, and Julian
Use the wrong one and risk damage to your reputation

So even the date is something unsure
Still the effort to gauge it is an effort pure
What is the time and what is the date
Again I ask, can anyone clearly state?

But when time certain is not of the essence
We employ the hourglass which defies obsolescence
Handy for egg cooking and gauging the passage of time
Even for the modern day its use is not a crime

And there are also simple timers we employ
For tracking work functions and things we enjoy
For comparing performances in athletic events
They measure overall time as well as segments

So the absolute time while not easily got
Is a goal we seek, a value not easily bought
Still we do our best to closely evaluate
Its approximate value, hour, minute, and date

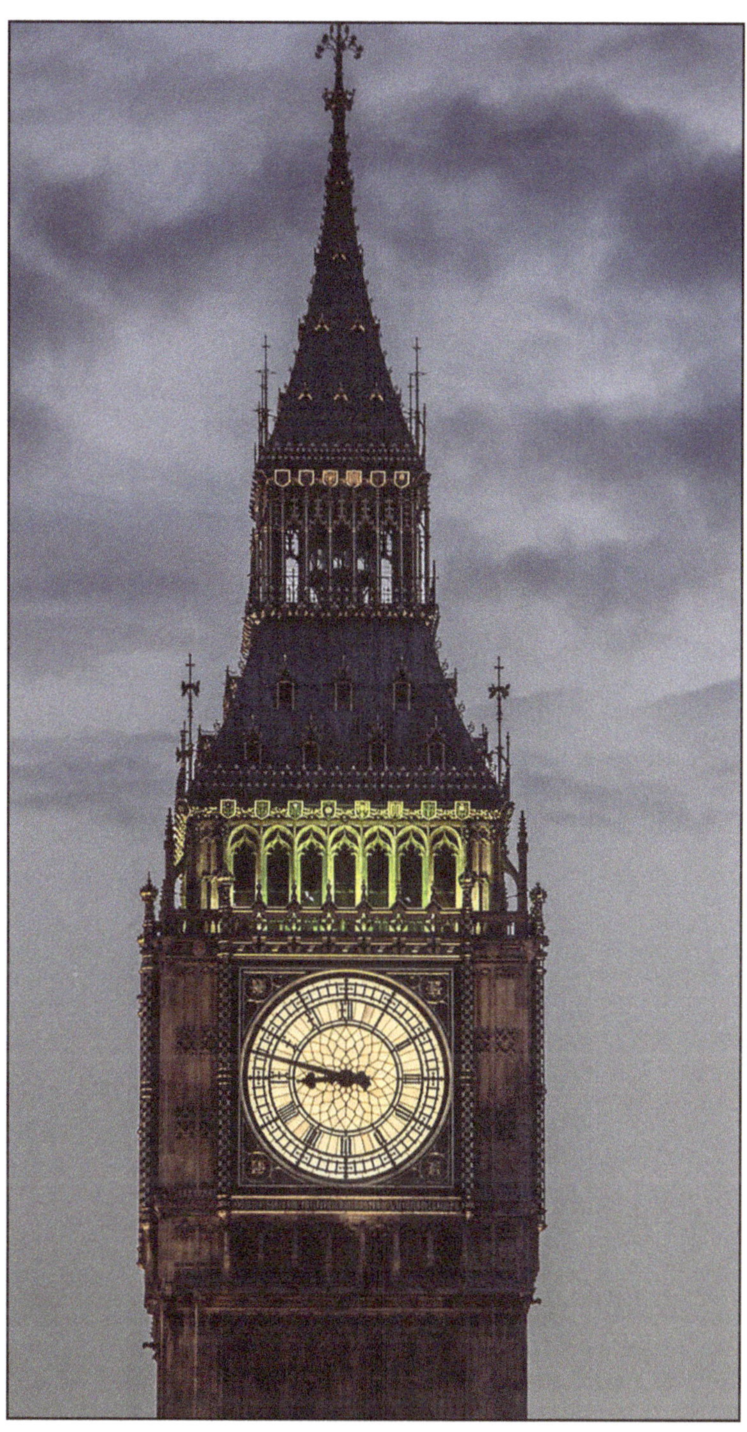

Big Ben

The Septuagenarian

In a week I'll turn seventy
In a case of superannuation
I'll try to use some levity
To make the best of the situation

As I morph into a septuagenarian
I try my best to remain calm
But I find I tend toward contrarian
And need to use reflection as a balm

So far I've managed to keep my wits
Despite attempts to forestall them
Despite the onset of the birthday blitz
Mere tree rings I will call them

Never thought I'd be this old
I'm amazed by it every day
For a pittance my youth was sold
I squandered it in many a way

I spend my days assaying the past
Spend little time on the future
If memory fails the past won't last
Memory rifts will need a suture

As I grow older I watch my diet
Look for vitamins, fiber and protein
Check for nutrients before I try it
There are dietary pitfalls unseen

I try to get myself some exercise
I do try each and every day
About healthy weight I fantasize
To attain it I try in every way

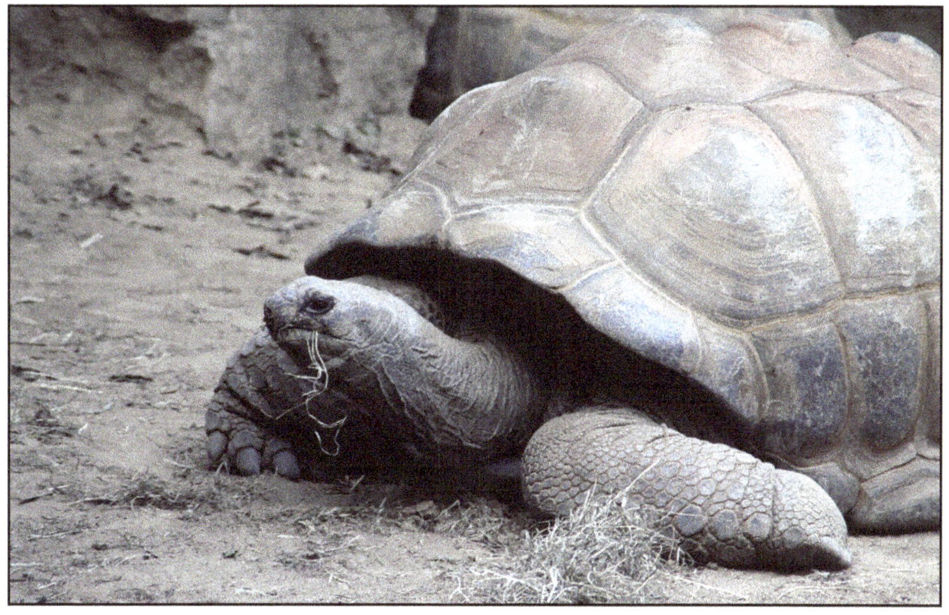

70 Ain't That Old

As I age I find that options do reduce
Fewer physical activities are possible
I begin to wear age as a strangling noose
That tightens making some things impossible

To stave off mental deficiency
I do my best at rhyming
I try to work with efficiency
I work hard on the timing

I try to choose my topics carefully
Yes, no fair subject to eschew
Sometimes I do it fruitfully
Other times it just won't do

Some works make it to the printer
Still others are simply thrown out
Not everyone turns out a winner
Some just make me want to pout

It does me good to have something
I'm happy to do each and every day
Sometimes the effort's worth nothing
Seems some days I've nothing to say

But there is something of worth
In trying writing everyday
Even when there's a dearth
Of worthwhile things to say

So for at least seventy more years
I'll try very hard to verbally vent
Try my best to stave off all the tears
Over where the first seventy went

Joe Smith

School Daze

This is a tale about education
Not meant to be a form of sedation
You may not find it very exciting
My hope is it will be enlightening

Education begins at an early age
When one learns that a little rage
Will get you fed sooner or later
Cry out or scream whichever is greater

Soon enough, then, it's off to preschool
Where subjects include the Golden Rule
Efforts are made to teach socialization
Results are subject to examination

Next come the primary grades
This is where the mistakes are made
New efforts made toward socialization
But comes a new factor, intimidation

Lessons include mastery of the alphabet
Sufficient time is allotted and yet
Some sad students fail to master
These basic concepts; a disaster

Learning takes place on the playground too
The student learns what to do and not do
Play along to get along is a central theme
The import of behaving like a part of a team

Maybe experience includes team sports
This depends on what the school supports
Games are played, it seems, of all sorts
Some even require specialized courts

Music, too, is introduced
The student's muse to seduce
Civics, maybe, and geography
Clubs appear, like photography

Glee clubs suddenly arrive on the scene
Even allowed when budgets are lean
An extension of efforts to teach musicality
An effort to promote harmony in all actuality

Mathematics increase in severity
Accompanied by a decrease in clarity
Some students, though, seem to thrive
While others only manage to survive

Then comes eighth grade graduation
Changing the student's situation
Plans for the future begin to unfold
When effort and guidance are controlled

Next up, application may be made
To schools where foundations are laid
For collegiate work that's anticipated
In the event academics aren't dissipated

Further progress is made towards socialization
Which since grade school has been in incubation
Societal requirements reflected in such as dances
Leads many a student to budding romances

Classes include introduction to polemics
And other new realms of academics
New methods of development are found
Best for those who are soon college bound

School rivalries do abound
Friendly enemies soon are found
Battles fought in the name of games
Passion and violence execution tames

Finally comes another graduation
For some this is school cessation
Still others must go on to college
Seeking as they do, more knowledge

College can prove quite the chore
Offering, as it does, majors galore
Each course with its own syllabus
To show its contents so rigorous

Social societies seem to set the stage
For long term relationships all the rage
Fraternities, sororities, professional clans
All help to contribute to future plans

Working toward matriculation
Relying on studious causation
The student exerts his erudition
Where facts reaffirm his own cognition

After all the arts and science
With many facts held in abeyance
Students approach another graduation
This time, for most, a fixed situation

Now for some comes graduate school
Where with the higher theories they'll duel
Success here can surely be supplanted
Where drop out rates are plainly granted

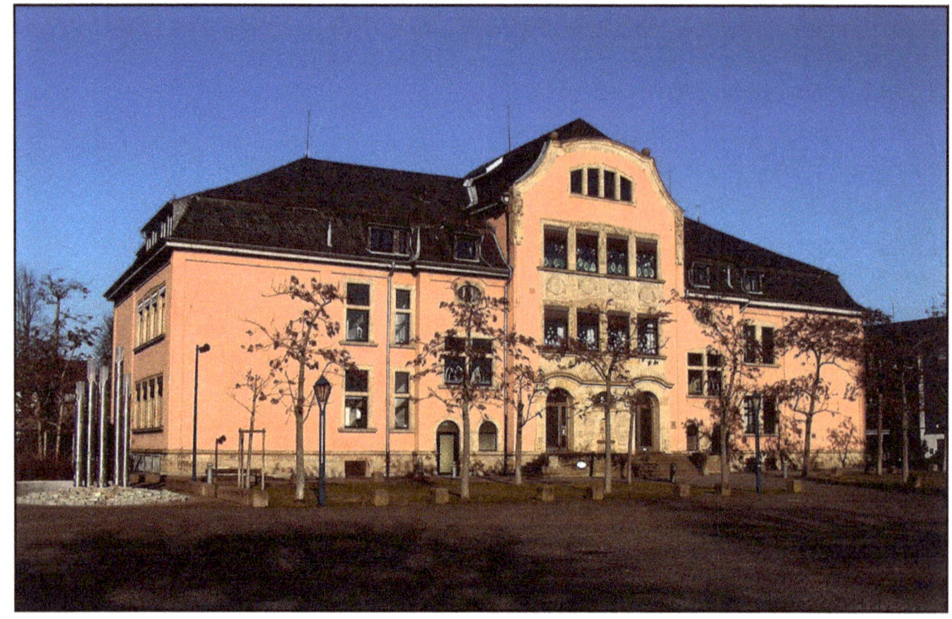

School Building

Once the school daze has dissipated
The move to the real world is overrated
The best advice I have ever heard
Was "stay in school" as the final word

In Anticipation of Procrastination

I was going to do some writing
About some thoughts I had
It's really not that exciting
Despite the lines I'd add

I thought about the times
When I would write right
Lines that end in rhymes
New passions to ignite

But then I got myself to thinking
What these lines should be about
And from the task I started shrinking
It was hard to get the words out

And so I started struggling
With each line and every verse
With the words I was juggling
Still the stanzas came out worse

So for a while I was committed
To cranking out the nouns and verbs
As long as inspiration permitted
Me to generate some pleasing blurbs

But I wasn't sure I would finish
This the latest rhyme of mine
Seemed something would diminish
My work despite invested time

It seems safe to say I was distracted
From the words as I would choose them
Something in my head detracted
From the words, it seems, I'd lose them

And still I continued in my search
For the appropriate word choice
Yet I was somehow left in the lurch
Thoughts were left without a voice

Then I began to doubt I'd finish
Despite my very strong exertion
Seems something would diminish
My attempts at word insertion

They say you shouldn't put off
That which you can do today
Advice at which I will not scoff
The piper's due his pay

But I just won't self criticize
If I don't finish this poem today …

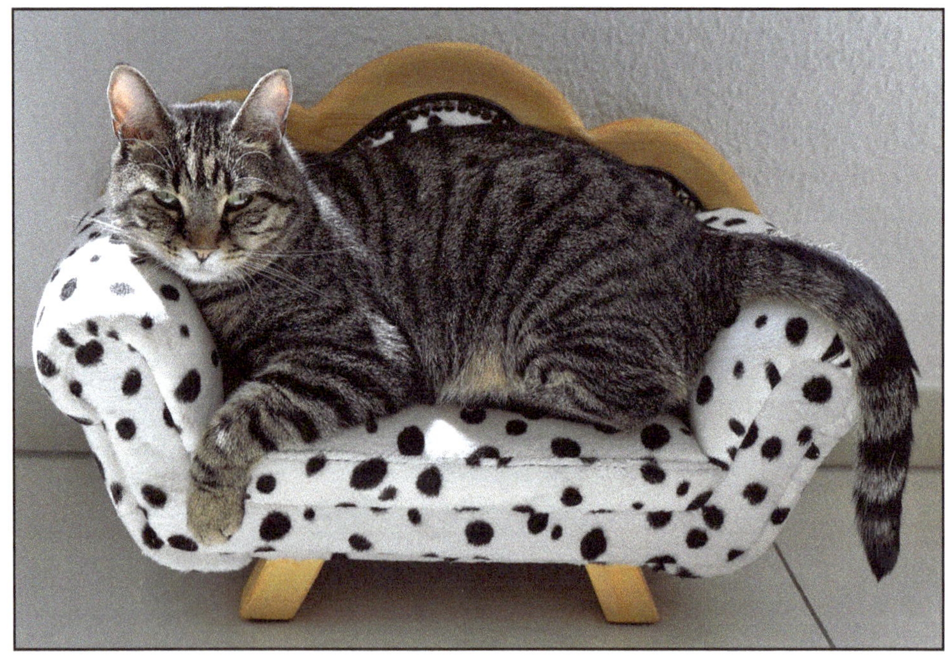

More Important Things To Do Today

Joe Smith

Only a Memory

We were 16 years old
I was anything but bold
I looked at her in total awe
Waiting for a relationship thaw

She was slender and petite
Her hair short and neat
With dimples in each cheek
I beheld her mystique

Her company I came to crave
But I was anything but brave
I couldn't make unwanted advances
Had to bide my time, take my chances

I bought her a small cameo ring
To me it was a special thing
She asked me though,"What does it mean?"
A question I had not foreseen

I shifted my weight and started to stammer
The blood at my temples started to hammer
"It means whatever you want"
I tried not to be too blunt

For her I had taken a chance
Set aside my fear and learned how to dance
Saved up my money to buy her a gift
Giving it to her gave my spirits a lift

If only I had the nerve to kiss her
Then perhaps I wouldn't miss her
But all the time I was so nervous
My reticence did me no service

Many years later, to my surprise
Her name in a conversation did arise
She told a friend she liked and missed me
Oh only, if only, she had just kissed me

If she had just done what I couldn't do
We might have turned into we two
But as it was we were both too uncertain
And so rang down love's opaque curtain

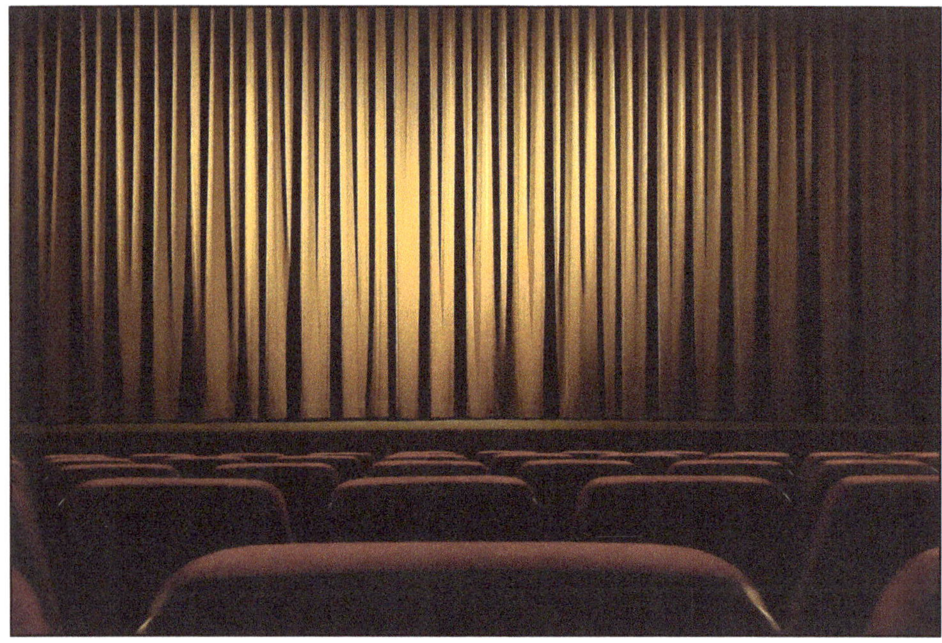

Nothing To See Here

Joe Smith

Marinading Memories

As time goes by I find that I
Value my memories more each day
And I find no matter how I try
I can't get enough of them to stay

But for those that do choose to stay
There seems to be a transformation
And so I guess what I'm trying to say
Is it helps to engage in some memory flirtation

As time passes they seem more substantial
They become somehow less ethereal
Take on a nature that is more consequential
They seem to become "solid" material

As I flipped through a family album today
I saw many pictures of things from the past
When I took the pictures I thought things would stay
I didn't realize that, in fact, they wouldn't last

Things like houses, cars, and various collections
Things that over time slipped through my grasp
But I've found somehow time brings recollections
That, if you let it, your mind is able to solidly clasp

These recollections take the form of marinated memories
Each with distinctive sights, touch, smell, and taste
With a little effort these sensations mature into reveries
Time spent pondering these elements isn't a waste

The lost items are replaced by these memories
Which morph into "things" that exist on their own
You no longer miss so dearly these treasuries
Your mind manufactures replacements to loan

But I should take time to issue a warning
These methods don't apply to the dearly departed
Don't try to solidify memories of mourning
Such efforts are not advised for the fainthearted

These marinated memories are of things
They aren't intended to represent a person
The loss of loved ones forever stings
Unlike things, people memories can worsen

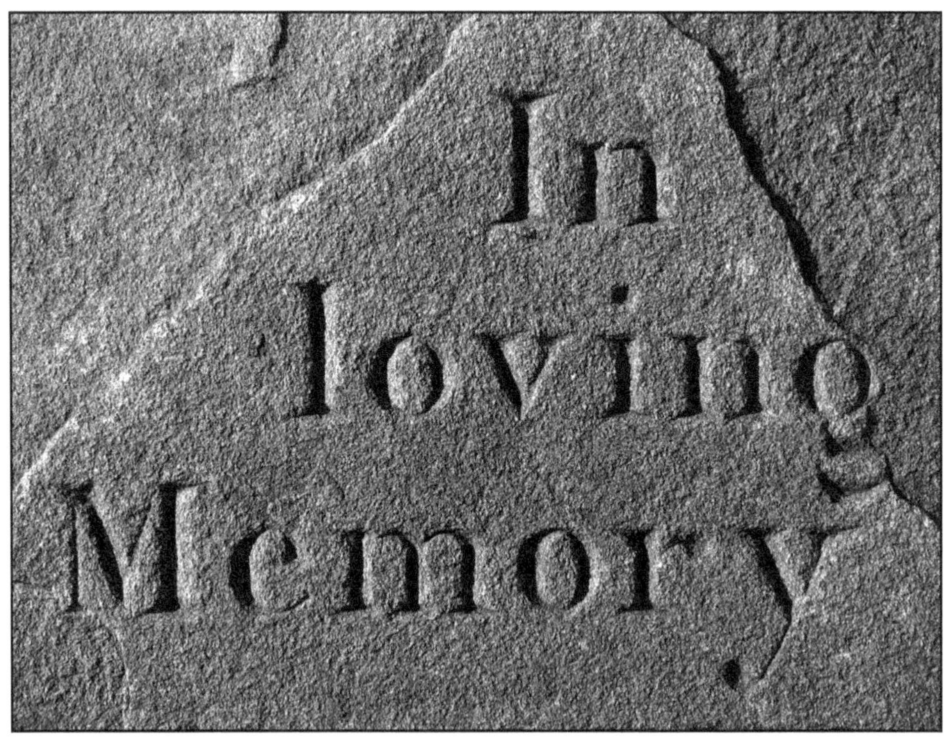

Handle With Care

Joe Smith

The Mad Mendicant

I knew a certain man
Much to my sorrow
Who rather than plan
Would much rather borrow

He'd even borrow the air that you breathe
He labored under no compunction
And while he made you slowly seethe
He was simply lacking in gumption

He once borrowed an item from me
And promised that he would return it
Polonius said, "neither borrower nor lender be"
It was a lesson, I should have learned it

When it came to borrowing he was a master
There was nothing he wouldn't ask for
Items small or large, all were sought after
It turned out his visage I began to deplore

After a while, he grew even bolder
He eventually asked to borrow the rent
There was no favor he'd mind that you shoulder
Just as long as what you had, to him, you lent

He'd borrow clothes right under your nose
Brand new or used, he sure paid no mind
From out of my closet the best garb he chose
He'd "borrow" from you until he stole you blind

More than a borrower he was a mendicant
Living off nothing but the generosity of others
Living life lazy and wholly impenitent
Pride in ownership, in others, he smothered

At one point it seems he needed a procedure
One that required the transplant of a vital part
You'd have thought he was having a seizure
As he proceeded to tear all his benefactors apart

He demanded the loan of a lobe of a liver
This was a loan he could never repay
His friends knew that he was no giver
But they decided to help anyway

So despite his underlying ingratitude
His friends finally decided to draw lots
To see who would help despite the attitude
Of the mad mendicant who called the shots

And so finally a victim was selected
Considered to be the perfect match
Slim chance the tissue would be rejected
Steps were taken with all due dispatch

The operation was considered a success
The mad mendicant fully recovered
He was surely no longer in distress
And still no gratitude was discovered

So swiftly the years did go by and time did pass
And nothing about the mad mendicant changed
There were hopes and prayers for transference, but alas
His appreciation and consideration remained deranged

And finally, there came about his passing
Most of his relationships had been estranged
On the nature of his friends he had been trespassing
But still it came time for his funeral to be arranged

As you can imagine it was a simple affair
No great expense was thought necessary
Sadly, only a few hearty souls were there
Only the most generous souls helped to bury

Very few attended as I have previously stated
To keep expenses down, it was a cremation
Of course all the flowers were donated
Fervent prayers were said to stave off damnation

After the ceremony, a trip to the columbarium
It was doubtful that this was the right location
Some thought he belonged in a museum
Installation in a columbarium, above his station

Still to the columbarium his ashes were finally taken
But there a final issue arose which had to be resolved
One which, when carefully considered, couldn't be mistaken
His many debts spiritual and material couldn't be dissolved

So was affected the matter of the memorial plaque
It was difficult to determine what it should say
It wasn't expected that he would be coming back
So there was the matter of who would pay

Even in death the mad mendicant was a bum
He, of course, once again failed to pay his own way
What he was differed little from what he'd become
Yes, it was difficult to decide what his memorial should say

And once again lots were drawn
From among his benefactors
In true regard for days bygone
A writer was chosen from his detractors

And the loser wrote

"While the mention of him lead to dental gnashes
And thoughts of him caused guts churned
The accumulation of his own ashes
Was the first thing that he ever urned"

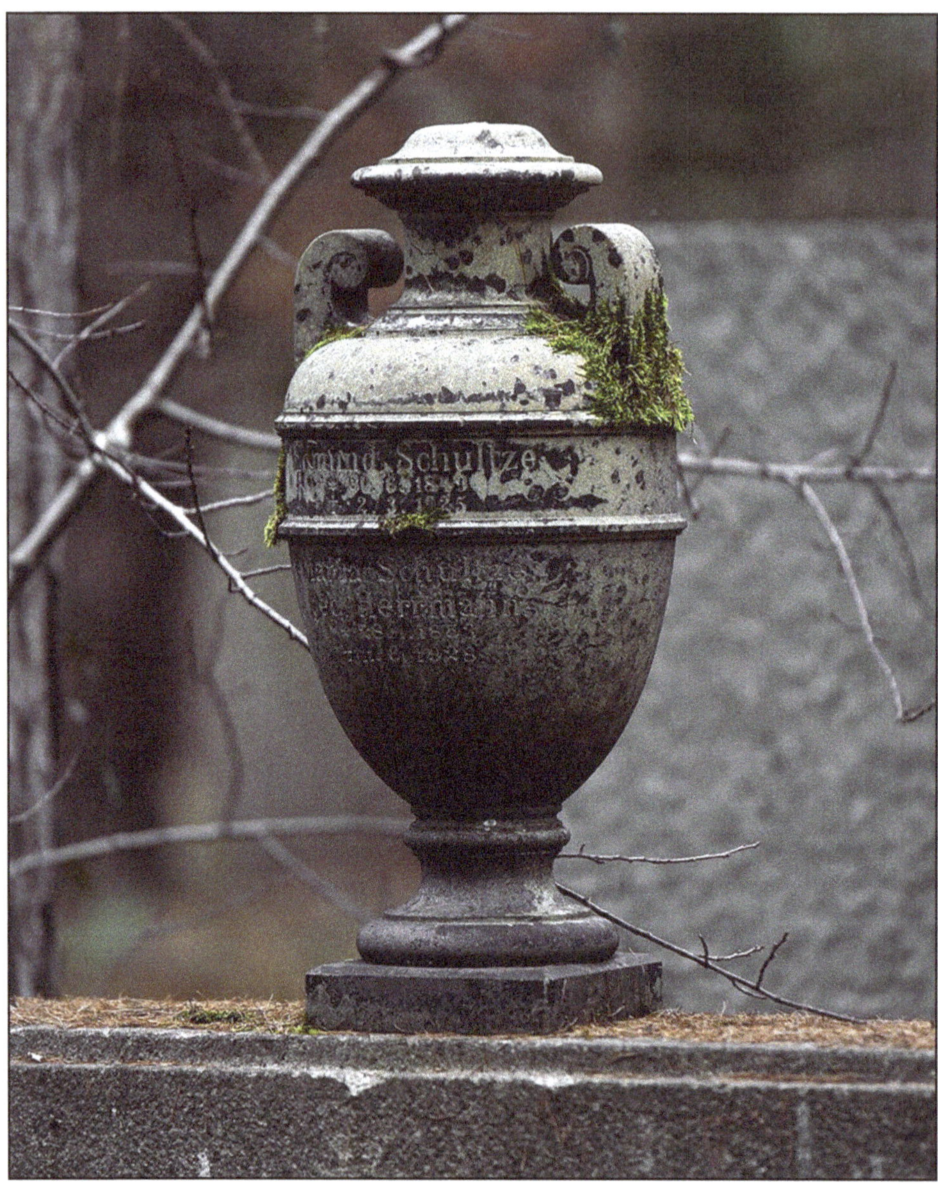

Funerary Urn

Broken Connection

Now she's gone and I can't reach her
In many ways she was my teacher
Showed me how to live life well
Instead of living like life's hell

Where she went I'll never know
I sit and wait, feel the fondness grow
Which part of her is the part that's real
The part I Know or the part I Feel?

That distinction's why I'm not sure
If my logic's clear, intentions pure
It's that problem of mine I'm thinking of
What exactly is what some call love?

Broken Connection

Crazy Comments Concerning Car Colors

I've noticed of late
Cars looking great
There's something new
I'm sure of it too
The change is the paint
The colors quaint
The many blues
Of electric hues
50 shades of gray
Are out today
Choose battleship
By color chip
Or gunmetal
On one please settle
Red Rose is fine
Let ruby shine
Even the beige
Is of a new gauge
And the greens
Have a new sheen
And there's a new yellow
It's very mellow
Of course there's white
And that's still alright
But now there is pearlescent
Of all the whites it is the essence
Glossy or flat
Shiny or matte
All the new tints
Of new days hint
And I must say that I like them

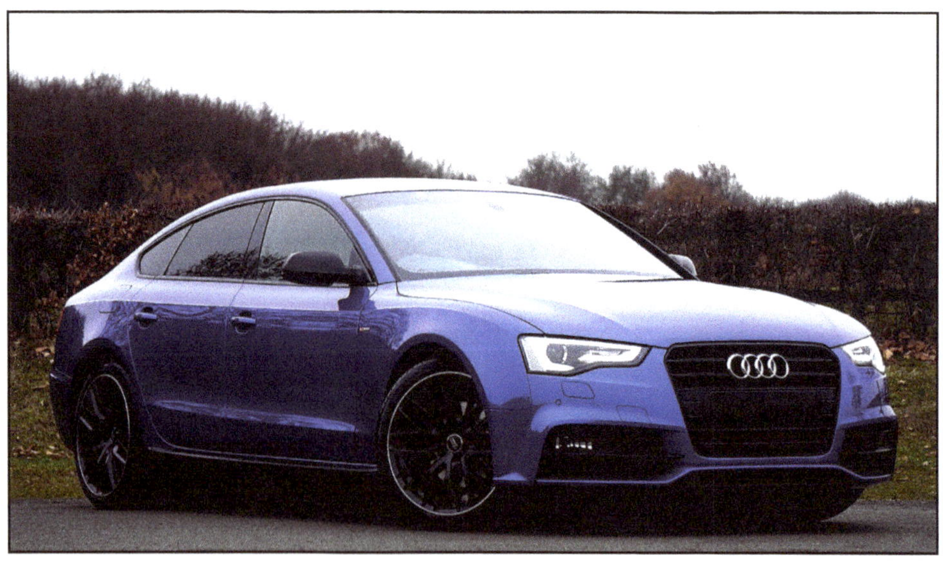

Beautiful Blue

Joe Smith

Early Morning Rising

I rose early, got out of bed
Thoughts were swirling in my head
Couldn't decide which one to deal with
Which to ignore and which to get real with

As I sit here somewhat quizzical
With thoughts of the metaphysical
I wonder why I cannot sleep
These thoughts into my mind do creep

Sometimes when I can't sleep
My mind wades out into the deep
I have thoughts I don't understand
Some are simple, others grand

Most are brought on by dreams
Where the fact of the matter isn't what it seems
Which are false and which are real
I can't tell by the way I feel

It's too early to make a call
Wondering if I will at all
Or will I keep this to myself
Wrap it up, put it on the shelf

Or maybe try to write it out
And neglect to give a shout
To anyone, anyone at all
Maybe I won't make the call

Sometimes, the thoughts, they bring me pain
But from consideration I don't abstain
I try my best not to sing a sad refrain
For fear these thoughts will come again

No, it is best that they be dealt with
For all the things that they'll be felt with
It is folly to let these lie
With these thoughts it's do or die

Bring them to their fair conclusion
Deal with them without delusion
Take advantage of early consideration
Don't wait for days of desperation

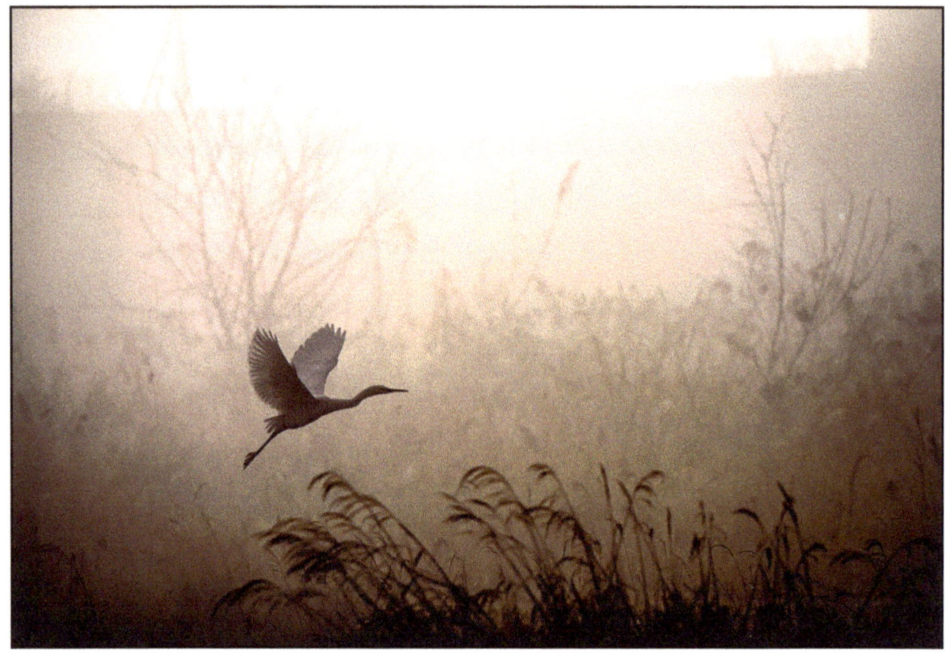

Never Regret Seeing The Egret Early In The Morning

Joe Smith

The Green Eyed Monster

Often known as jealousy
It's a trait you often see
Hunted down by Mr. Shakespeare
It's the object of consummate fear

Believed to come from too much bile
Turning the skin green, this feeling vile
It eventually invades each and every pore
Tries to choke off joy for evermore

Leads by needs to self destruction
Inch by inch due to false deduction
There's no winning this foul game
Often the truth it does defame

Starts off with a kind of yearning
Leads next into emotions burning
From false feelings the Monster's fed
His green eyes will soon see red

Habitually ignoring all that's tried and true
The Monster holds its breath 'til it turns blue
Eventually it becomes a rainbow raptor
Alluding each and every class of captor

Rings the death knell on many a romance
For fear of it, many decline to dance
Surveying possibilities with it's green eyes
Passion found in others it does despise

Many times it lies in wait
Twixt the poles of heaven's gate
Daring its victim to escape
While assuming yet another shape

From raptor to a snake it evolves
To reach the low down ones it solves
The problem of unique revenge
The slightest slight to avenge

The bite of the Monster is deadly
Its venom and malintent a medley
Comprised of slightly warped reason
Against fair play it commits high treason

The Monster is the king of wants
When shown the facts he only grunts
It bothers him not to deceive
Twisted logic he hopes you will perceive

The Green Eyed Monster will lie to you
He will tell you things that just aren't true
He'll make you want what you just can't own
He is master of the discontent he's sown

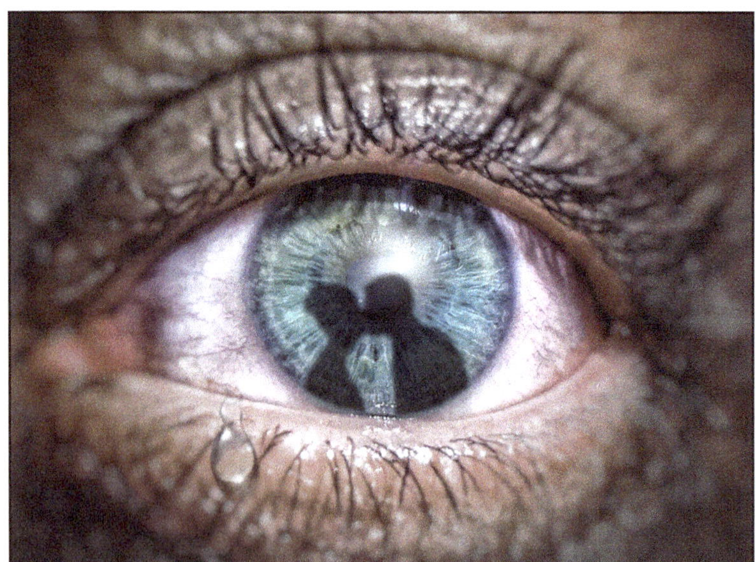

An Eye Of The Monster

Joe Smith

In Search of a Kind Word

I'm only just sitting here
My purpose isn't exactly clear
Trying to just sit and think
About a lexicographic link

This is mostly about my mood
In my own juices I have stewed
Trying my best to break out
Of this foul mood I've been about

Trying right now to find just the word
To change my outlook when it's heard
Looking now for that single thought
That happier times have finally brought

The more I think about this task
The more I think myself to ask
Could there be a magic word
That 'til now has not been heard

Or is there maybe an existing syllable set
That I have failed to employ as yet
Maybe a word with special properties
Or does my malevolent mind just tease

I think now into the distant past
To a friend of mine I knew at last
Who during a deep assay of the mind
Offered that her goal was children kind

She could affect the desired effect
For her children's mores she'd not neglect
She led them all with kindness ample
Yes I would say she was a fine example

Yes, in a conversation somewhat philosophical
Where thoughts were traded, though unofficial
From below the depths of thought there came
Her profession that kindness won the game

Her most fervent hope for her progeny
Was that they be simply kind you see
She thought that alone leads to happiness
And there's truth in her thought I must confess

For in being kind to other creatures
Kindness to ourselves soon features
The very best of being human
Other virtues soon to illumine

Kindness is true and tried
When universally applied
The magic sought soon is spied
When with openness it is allied

Kindness doled out in every case
Helps us soon to win the race
Thus kindness is the word I find
To help ease my worried mind

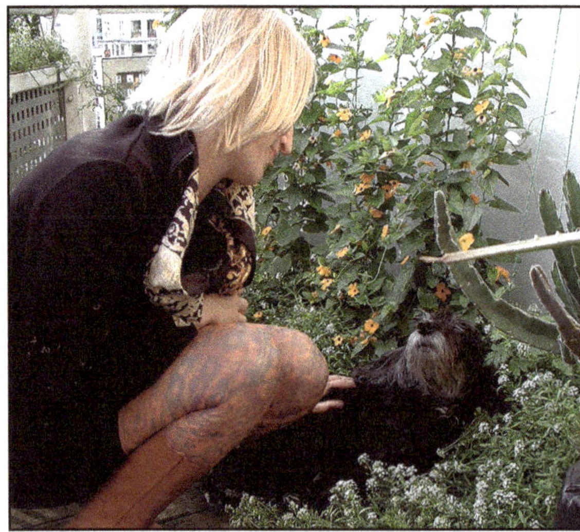

Kindness Can Be Shown
In A Host Of Ways

First Kiss

Every now and then
I remember when
I was a young man
When it all began

I went on my first date
I wasn't feeling great
I was feeling very shy
I was scared I won't deny

She was a tall slim beauty
I thought she felt a duty
To make me feel comfortable
And not quite so vulnerable

We had only recently met
But we made a fair duet
An athlete and a drummer
I expected nothing from her

But boy was I surprised
A feeling that I disguised
When suddenly she kissed me
As if she couldn't resist me

I had never been kissed before
Having had this one, I wanted more
To say the least I found it exciting
I found the whole situation inviting

We headed, then, to a dance
I felt as if I were in a trance
The kiss turned out to be just one feature
Of a magical night with this lovely creature

Years went by and we stayed together
I thought for a while it would last forever
But then she told me there was another
And she began to treat me like a brother

After awhile we grew apart
Odd it seemed, given our start
But after all this time I miss
The moment she gave me my first kiss

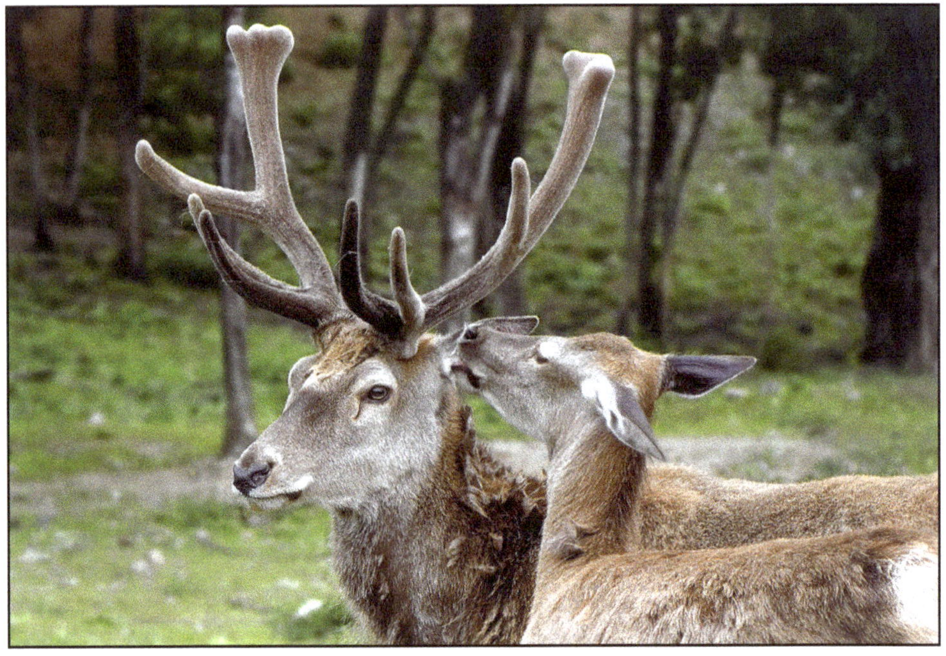

First Kiss?

Joe Smith

*Residential Redoubt**

This is a tiny tale about
My residential redoubt
About my personal fort
Where I am king of the court

It's a description of my retreat
Which I endeavor to keep very neat
I will tell you of some of my belongings
Which reflect my various longings

First on the list is the lighting
Something I find quite exciting
Incandescent and LED
So enlightening there for me

Now that at last we can see
I'll tell you of my new TV
Months go by and it's not on
Wouldn't miss it if it were gone

Except for use with the three players
Used as DVD and VHS purveyors
I hope some day to begin to view
My digital movies all the way through

Now my favorite item is my desk
Where I perform verbal burlesque
A common platform with a hutch
Where I write my poems and such

Sitting alone by the wall is my bed
Where I used to lay my head
It has since been deserted
And a recliner has been inserted

Next to the recliner is a leather love seat
The two together constitute a suite
The love seat is a great resting place
Does more than just take up space

Then there are three sets of shelves
That are attention grabbers in themselves
Holding hundreds of movies, tapes, and books
They surely deserve some extra looks

Centered in the living room space
Is a sound system, out of place
Seven hundred and seventy watts
It's high on my list of whatnots

It provides a host of acoustical treats
The sub woofer accentuates the beats
The system tends to analyze sounds
From its host of speakers life abounds

Within the fortress are several files
Standard and lateral, there are two styles
Letters, forms, and pictures they contain
Evidence and memories they maintain

Sitting about are family pictures
Presenting as they do, mental strictures
Of times gone by and opportunities missed
Pleasant memories as well as ill persist

Within the walls there is a kitchen
Though little used, I should mention
A cook top I plan one day to use
And in the ice box there are some clues

As to what I like, at times, to eat
For either a staple or as a treat
Some protein for the siege is nice
The vicious Vandals to entice

Of this there can be no doubt
I feel safe in my redoubt
I have sufficient survival supplies
More sustenance than you'd realize

My redoubt, you see, has but one door
More defenses required if there were more
Controlled access through this portal
Guaranteed for all but the immortal

There is, of course, a lock upon the door
To prevent likely theft, which I abhor
To thwart the efforts of a thieving hoarder
And to promote a general sense of order

And so within these walls I survive
With possessions protected I try to thrive
And so I reside here within my bastion
Living life simply, no plans for expansion

**Redoubt - a temporary or supplementary fortification*

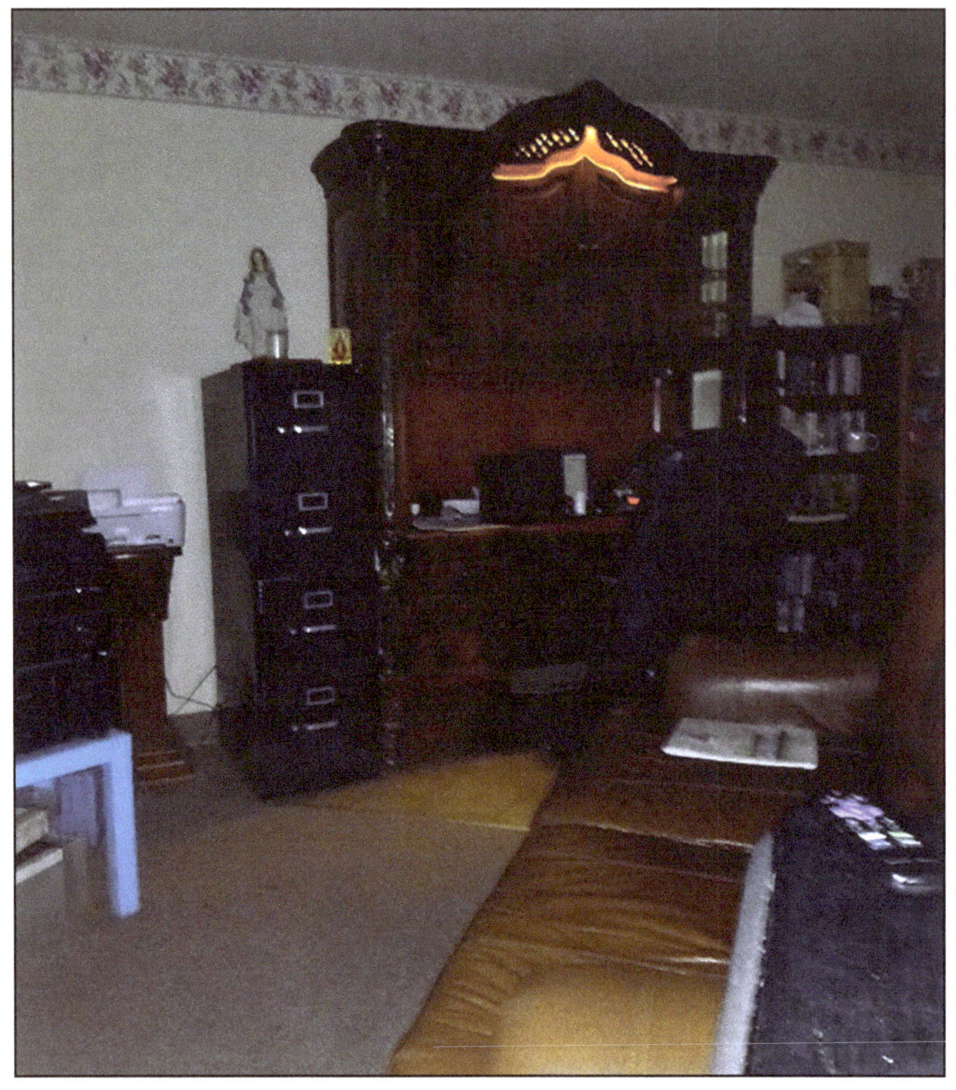

Redoubt

APPENDIX ONE

My Family

In this collection I refer to several of my siblings as being kind.
The word may seem overworked
except for the importance given this description
in the poem "In Search of a Kind Word"
The experience related therein helps to explain
my reliance on this word in describing my siblings.

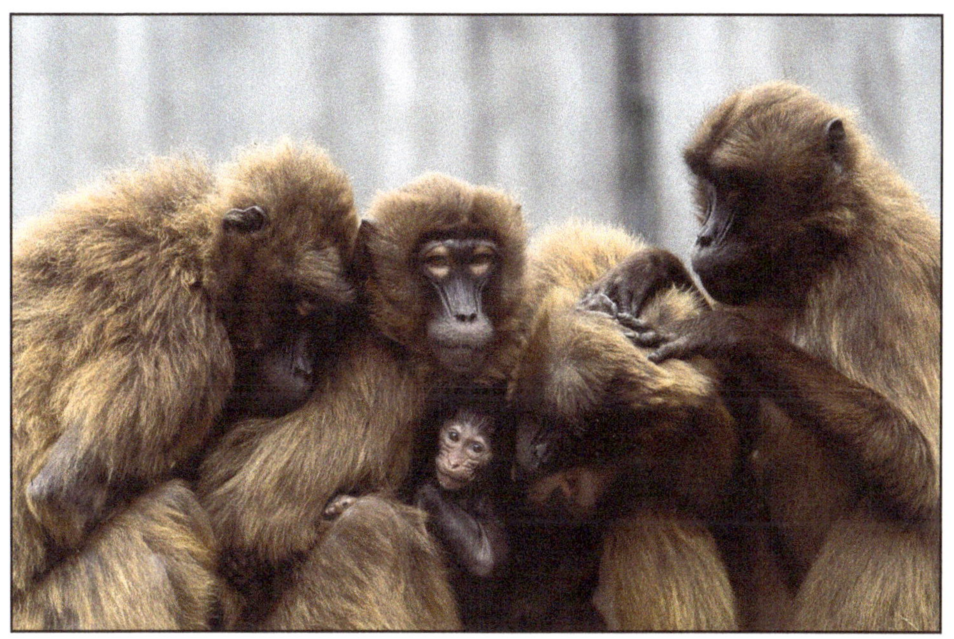

A Close Knit Family

*Echo**
(My Dad)

I hear your voice
Dear Daddy still
Not what I want
But what you will

There's no one else
I've truly trusted
To know what's right
And well adjusted

Every time I start to think
Your voice comes booming through
And even if I don't concur
I take your point of view

With troubled but single personality
I muddle through each day
Still your voice lends duality
To all I do and say

I wonder just what might have been
If I had had the choice
To listen to or no ear lend
To the sound of your tired voice

Yes, wonder just what might have been
If you hadn't been my father
Could I to you have been a friend?
Or would you even bother?

Each time I take my pen in hand
To try to write what's true
I know there's nothing quite as grand
As what your hands could do

I measure each and every man
Against the mark you made
And I know that I never can
Roll down the tracks you laid

As I sit here on Christmas Eve
I cannot help but wonder
About the voice that I will leave
Will it cause them to blunder?

Or will I have a voice at all,
A whisper, SHOUT, or scream
To lead my children down the hall
Away from all that's mean?

I love you, Dad, don't take offense
But this to me is clear
A voice that keeps them on the fence
Is what I truly fear

I'd rather in the end they know
That one voice is all they need
Secure in knowing they should go
Where their own voices lead

**Originally appeared in* Life Between The Poles, *included here to complete family presentation*

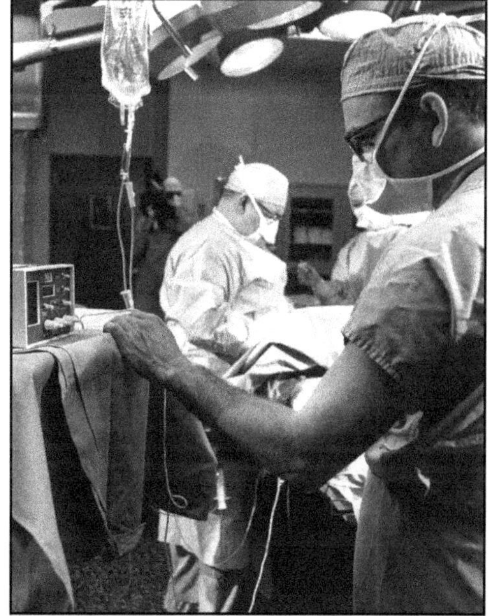

Dad Was A Surgeon

It Took Three Times

I really don't know how to write this
Because I don't know how I feel
This is not a tale of true bliss
But rather what is true and real

I truly loved my mother
As I hope you'll plainly see
But we challenged each other
Seldom let each other be

You see I was her problem child
Or so she once described me
But now I'm seventy and less wild
And wonder what she saw in me

I required much more of her time
Than my sisters and my brothers
She attended me nearly full time
Due to more surgeries than others

She very often reminded me
That I got more than all the rest
It was attention undesired you see
I tried to avoid it at my level best

But I was cursed with crossed eyes
And poor capacity to right them
And in these two facts the problem lies
I didn't try too hard to fight them

No I did my best to cooperate
With the doctors and the nurses
But fusion I could not perpetuate
My efforts led me to the inverses

And of course when it came to dentistry
My need for care was surely unmatched
I did not at any point engage in sophistry
Swelling caused normal care to be dispatched

So despite my best efforts to comply
With behavioral standards as laid out
My physical characteristics sought to defy
And difficult interactions then played out

There were times when I displeased her
Because I didn't know what a word meant
She thought I was trying to tease her
When I asked her on a word to comment

This happened to me more than one time
And the events remain seared in my mind
If she were a judge I would have done time
Lack of knowledge would put me in a bind

It was these events that led me to feign lexicography
The misunderstandings so strongly I did lament
Even more than my beloved discography
I learned the importance of what a word meant

Over the years I learned a great deal from my mother
About architecture, antiques, literature, and art
But, I wish I had had the literary appetite of my brother
In addition to avoiding misunderstandings, he got smart

When it came time to go away to college
To my surprise she hugged and kissed me
I can't say I knew how to acknowledge
The fact that she might really miss me

Years later when my family was California bound
We stopped by my parents house to say good-bye
I returned to retrieve an item I'd forgotten, I found
And was amazed to find my mother having a cry

Again, I was surprised at this reaction
I had expected to see a sigh of relief
But instead there was this odd distraction
That she was crying was beyond my belief

I was gone for two years when my Dad had his stroke
I returned home alone to see him one last time
As I watched Mom nurse him something in me awoke
I saw in her compassion for once in her lifetime

But I now know it was there all along
In raising ten children it surely was there
That I couldn't see it I now know was wrong
To let misunderstandings hide it was unfair

Four years would pass before I returned to home base
The occasion was the imminent death of my brother
And once again my mom nursed a familial case
And she attended his needs as could no other

During my visit my brother went up the stairs
But it was obvious he couldn't manage alone
So I helped him up and Mom climbed up unawares
I would break down and cry, thinking I was on my own

Once I got my brother into the bed
My mother came to me and held me
This time her touch I didn't dread
Her love somehow upheld me

Sadly I only saw her once again
Before she went away for good
And though it all involved such pain
I felt about my mother as I should

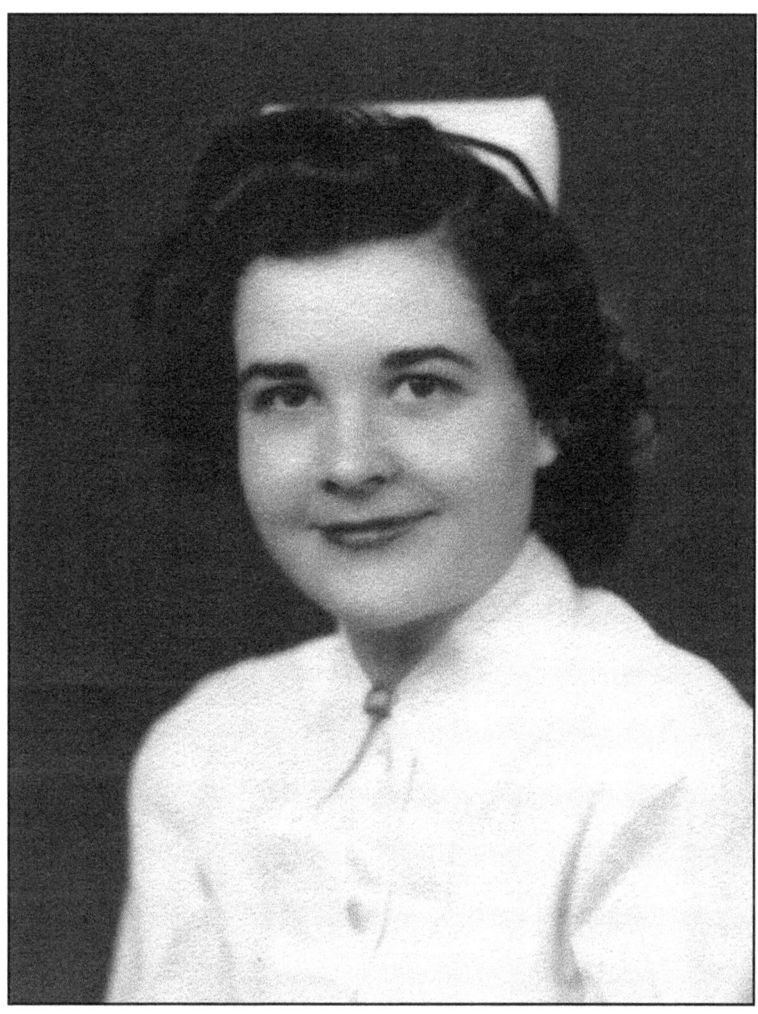

Mom Was A Nurse

Leader of the Pack
(Ruthie)

I was twelve years old before I knew
Her name was not Ruthelen
That's when I finally got a clue
Her real name was Ruth Helen

She was the oldest of us ten children
And by necessity became our leader
Her rise to the position wasn't sudden
As straw boss you couldn't beat her

(I add these 2 stanzas at my own peril)
When we were children we often fought
We went at it typically with both barrels
She always won, a win I couldn't have bought

During one of these spats she told me
A thing I'll never forget to embody
"I have more muscle in the back of my leg
Than you have in your whole body"

She was wise beyond her years
Truly a font of knowledge
From among all of her peers
She won scholarships to college

One was to Vanderbilt University in Tennessee
Another to Lady of the Lakes in Texas, don't you see
But she chose neither, in the end, though they were free
Instead she stayed at home and took good care of me

Well that wasn't the only reason she stayed
There certainly were other factors to be considered
Of course there were other pipers to be paid
With responsibilities her life was littered

She was always at the top of the list
I marveled at her composure
She was a National Merit Finalist
Thus she had her fair share of exposure

She had experience considerable
She did everything first, of course
She blazed the trail happy or miserable
She did nothing requiring remorse

She taught us to survive a car wreck
She did it in very elegant style
She very nearly broke her neck
She suffered a broken clavicle for awhile

Even now I have a faint memory
Of her transposing musical notes
From a typical sheet music repository
To the fingering each note denotes

This helped in learning the baroque recorders
Which Dad had given to us all
She was simply following Dad's orders
But the exercise in my eyes made her tall

She was very often the child in charge
A responsibility she gladly accepted
She thereby lived her life very large
Though officiousness she rejected

When I became a teen, and somewhat of a louse
She became even somewhat kinder to me
She drove me to my girlfriend's house
Blinders she wore; she couldn't see the real me

Many times she picked me up at work
Many times she dropped me off
She even came and picked me up, a jerk
When in a hot tempered rage I'd run off

One time when I was 16 years old
She let me drive her car
Thus she had acted very bold
Though we didn't go very far

She even sat in the back seat
And let my girlfriend sit in the front
I always thought that was pretty neat
But, the whole thing was just a stunt

As time passed she did more memorable things for me
Like the time she nursed my oncoming hepatitis
She gave me a heating pad for my back, wouldn't let me be
It was things like this that I feel helped to unite us

When I finally left home with my brother
We moved into an adjacent apartment
To my sister who'd been like a mother
Ours was just an auxiliary compartment

We spent half our time at her place
She often fed us and entertained us
I don't know how she kept up the pace
She did nothing less than sustain us

And I can't speak of my sister
Without mentioning Ken
He was always with her
Yes he's with her now as he was then

They will soon be married fifty years
They were together long before that
Each one the other simply reveres
And in that time a daughter they begat

Ken has always been good to me
He's been quick to provide information
About devices mostly new to me
He's been helpful in many a situation

He too provided transportation
Way back in the day
He required no explanation
And did it without pay

I rely on his wealth of knowledge
He's helped me out more than once
(Among other things he taught in college)
Without making me feel like a dunce

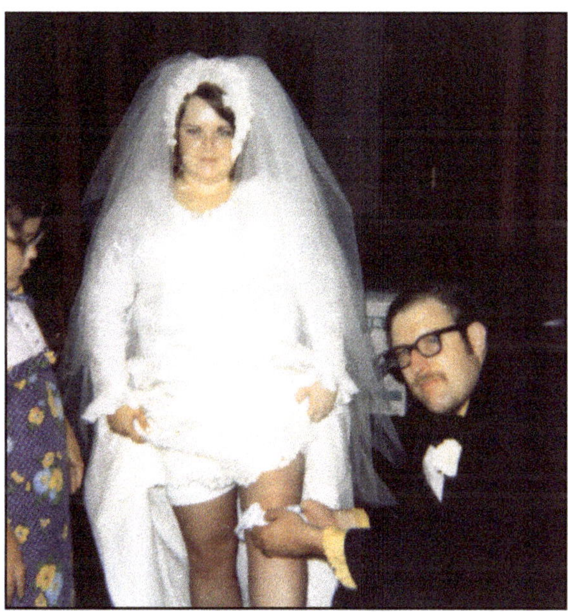

Ruth Helen and Kenny
On Their Wedding Day
- 1972

Quick Vic (Victor)

It's time I wrote a line or two
About my oldest brother
To finally give him his is due
He, too, is a credit to our mother

When he was about twelve years old
He had a paratrooper bike accident
The bike just opened at the fold
And quickly down he went

He had had a bad concussion
Of that there could be no doubt
No need for further discussion
Mom knew what she was talking about

I don't know why I recall this
Surely there were other things
Though of all the things to befall us
This one my memory bell rings

My fondest memories of Vic
Surround his penchant for drag racing
He is a talented mechanic
In our town known for its horse racing

Victor had a knack
For building a fast car
He took it to the track
And soon became a star

He won several trophies
Of that there is no doubt
I came to know all of these
As he would set them out

What I know for sure of Vic
He was completely car crazy
He was also very quick
And was anything but lazy

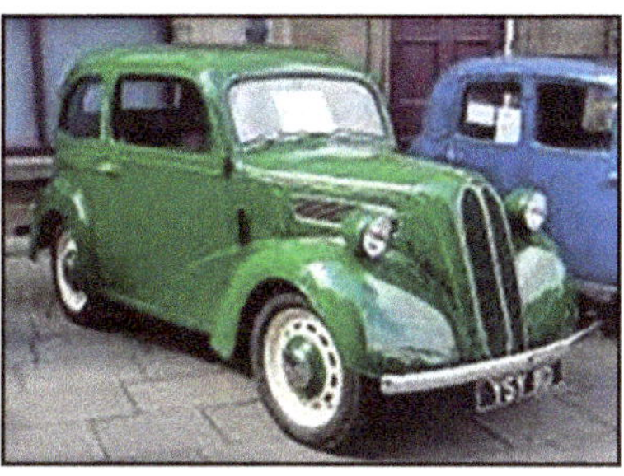

1952 Anglia

Of all the cars that he owned
The one I liked the best
Was a 1952 Anglia
It outshone all the rest

Because of what he knew
And he surely shared this knowledge
I was often exposed to
A veritable car college

To this day, I have my first choices
The '32 and '55 Chevys and the '40 Ford
He gave to all of these cars voices
That spoke in ways that couldn't be ignored

One year we took a very rare vacation
In an old borrowed modified school bus
That had traveled across our whole nation
As it turned out Vic's aptitude was a plus

You see my dad was pretty short
And had very short legs to match
The trip we almost had to abort
Because he couldn't push in the clutch

But Victor came up with a plan
That involved mounting blocks on the pedal
As it turned out Dad was a plan fan
And assigned Victor the problem to settle

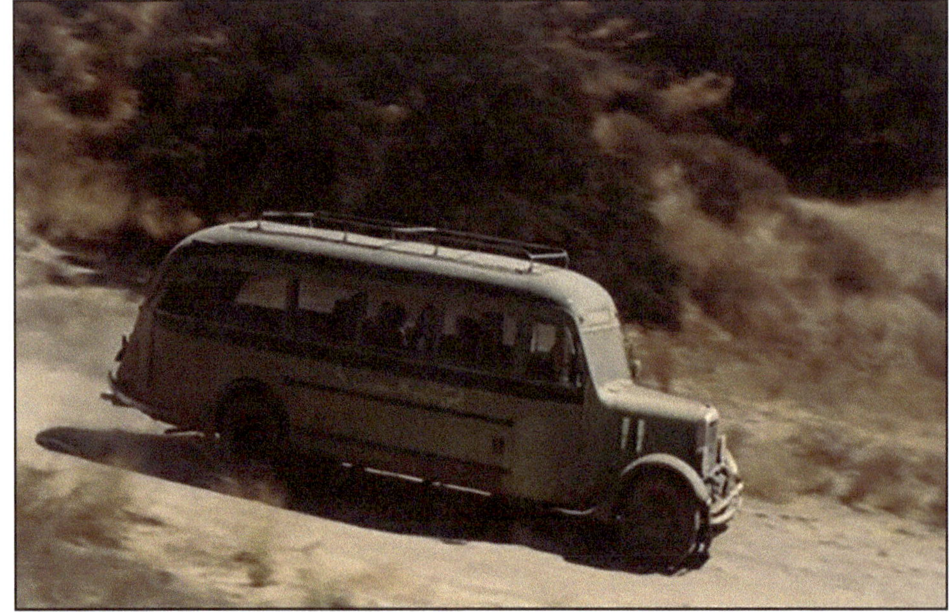

1933 GMC Bus

Writing this now I'm relying
On a memory fifty plus years old
Thus this may cause some denying
Of the tale that I have told

Of the plan to add the block I am certain
Less sure is the actual execution
For the veracity of the tale I accept the burden
At the risk of damage to my reputation

But in my mind I see the block
Mounted to the clutch pedal
But, of course, there is no lock
On my poor powers mental

But of all the things he did
This one I liked the best
He joined the Navy and heaven forbid
He operated heavy equipment with finesse

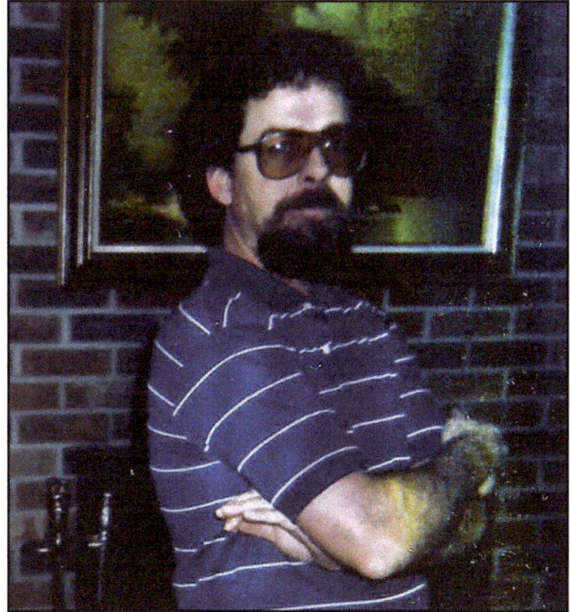

Victor Ulysses Smith

In the country of Morocco
He did his "A School" thing
While he missed his old Bultaco
He did heavy equipment handsprings

I have but one great regret
When it comes to my oldest male sibling
And that's that I never bet
Or saw him at his best, drag racing

I'm sorry if mistakes I'd trade
In writing this review I've made
As time goes by our memories fade
As into the past our minds do wade

Brother You Can Drive My Car
(Dennis Jameson)

I want to write a poem
But don't know where to start
Subject matter alludes me
And I struggle with this art

I thought I'd write about my brother
'Cause He's been so kind to me
There's simply been no other
Whose meant so much to me

I always admired his accomplishments
It seems there is nothing he can't do
I write this now without embellishments
Believe me when I claim each word I say is true

There are so many examples
I could provide to prove my point
But I'll just provide some samples
With his victories I will anoint

When we were mere boys at home
He joined the baseball little league
Not only did the bases he roam
But he played a part in the game's intrigue

He wound up becoming pitcher
In a game that to him was new
He made my life much richer
By being a role model too

Later he became an altar boy
So I became one too
All my effort I had to employ
To learn the Latin for my debut

Later he took on another role
As assistant to the music director
He turned thumbs down on my vocal goal
He simply acted as choir ejector

But there came a day when I realized
That he was right in his decision
I heard a tape of my voice digitized
And I knew he was right in my excision

And then there was his music
A science I could never master
A talent that was, for me, therapeutic
Bound my psychic wounds in healing plaster

Later he gave me more reasons for adulation
He learned to play the Sousaphone
And taught himself the guitar before graduation
He entertained me with our favorite tones

And while I have the chance
Let me tell you of one of his favors
He had his girlfriend teach me to dance
Which resulted in hours of pleasure to savor

I was just sixteen years old
And he was two years older
He took a step so bold
Almost too bold to shoulder

He was always loaning me things
Not the least of which was his car
I felt as if I'd grown wings
I was able to go near and far

Even work didn't interfere with his kindness
He'd let me use that car throughout the day
It was as if towards my defects he had a blindness
And even for gas he would not let me pay

To this day I don't understand
Why he took this risk with me
And why he didn't demand
A similar favor don't you see

I love all my brothers and sisters
Of which there are quite a few
But Dennis earned some blisters
By all the things for me he did do

I owe an honest attempt
To complete this exercise
Yes, for the full complement
Of my family, both gals and guys*

** This was the first of the sibling poems I wrote.*

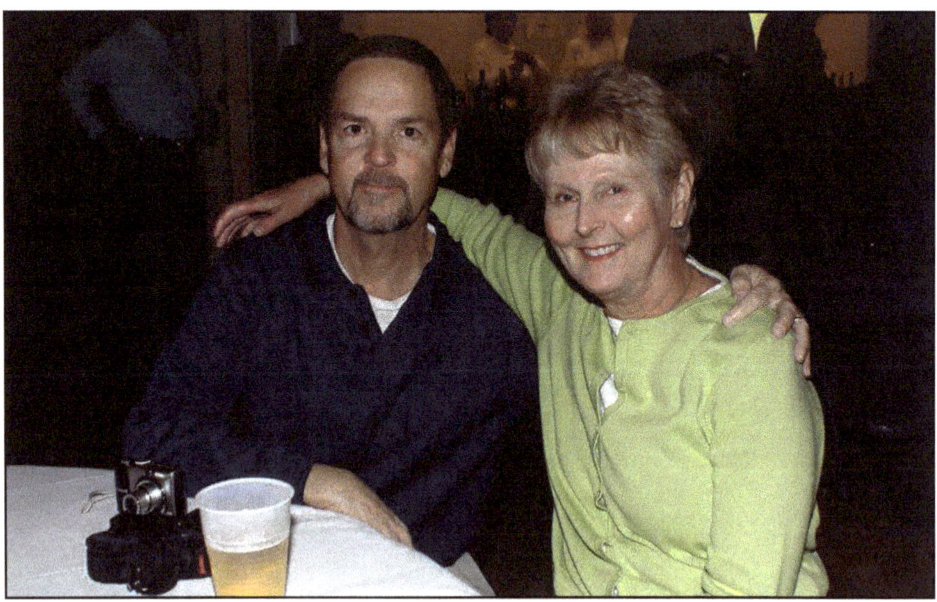

Dennis Was A Research Chemist
Seen Here With His Wife Rhonda

Kirby Louis Bernard Thomas Smith

The purpose of this work is to acquaint you
With another brother of mine
An accurate picture of him I will paint you
And in it I'll just let him shine

Of my brothers he was the smallest
But his name was by far the longest
And although he wasn't the tallest
Pound for pound he was the strongest

Kirby, it seems, was a mesomorph
He easily packed on muscle
I myself am an endomorph
For me weight loss is a tussle

But while I was living on a low cal diet
Kirby read in bed and drank cokes
While he looked diet compliant
I was the butt of fat people jokes

When school began intramural wrestling
Kirby found himself competing
With those composing the first string
In fact his weight class he was sweeping

From his earliest days he was an animal lover
He constantly read all about them
There was no species he didn't cover
As a source of animal info he was a gem

He hatched some duck eggs he found
Using a bun warmer on a stove pilot light
His plan turned out to be very sound
The ducklings hatched out all right

The ducklings imprinted on him
They followed wherever he went
Chances of losing them were slim
To care for them he was hell bent

He read voraciously of the Coturnix Quail
He decided that he would try to raise some
When it came to animals he'd never fail
He read too much about them to be dumb

He started with five: four hens and one male
Ended up with hundreds when he was done
From the five, yes hundreds would hale
So many there wasn't room for another one

These birds lay an egg each day
In an incubator he would hatch them
You couldn't keep the population at bay
If they got loose you couldn't catch them

That was just one poultry project
I recall particularly one more
It involved a guinea hen prospect
His fowl friends he did so adore

In addition to these fowl pets
He had several nice four footed friends
The best of them all, my memory begets
Was Liebchen, a St. Bernard girlfriend

We worked together at a florist
While there he was patient with me
He might have preferred life in the forest
To listening to stories from me

When I was a freshman in college
He was a year ahead of me
We went there to obtain knowledge
But back home was where I'd rather be

During the second semester
I was feeling quite sad and alone
He let me move in with him
Again, my stories he didn't bemoan

I have still a vague notion
Or perhaps it was only a dream
Of Kirby crocheting without emotion
While studying, or so it seems

At any rate he certainly has talent
As exhibited by my new afghan
Which he crocheted for an aunt
Who passed away soon after he began

It is one of my most prized possessions
I use it each and everyday
It certainly makes good impressions
Or at least that's what my friends say

But of all his qualifications
The one I admire the most
Is his encyclopedic conflations
Of which he does not boast

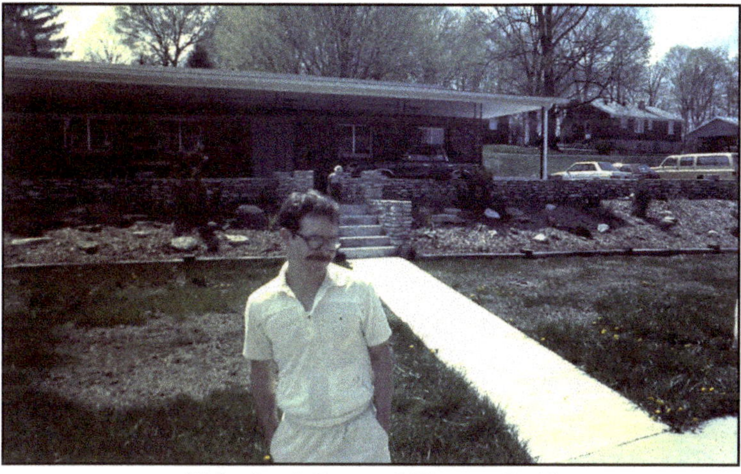

Kirby Louis Bernard Thomas Smith

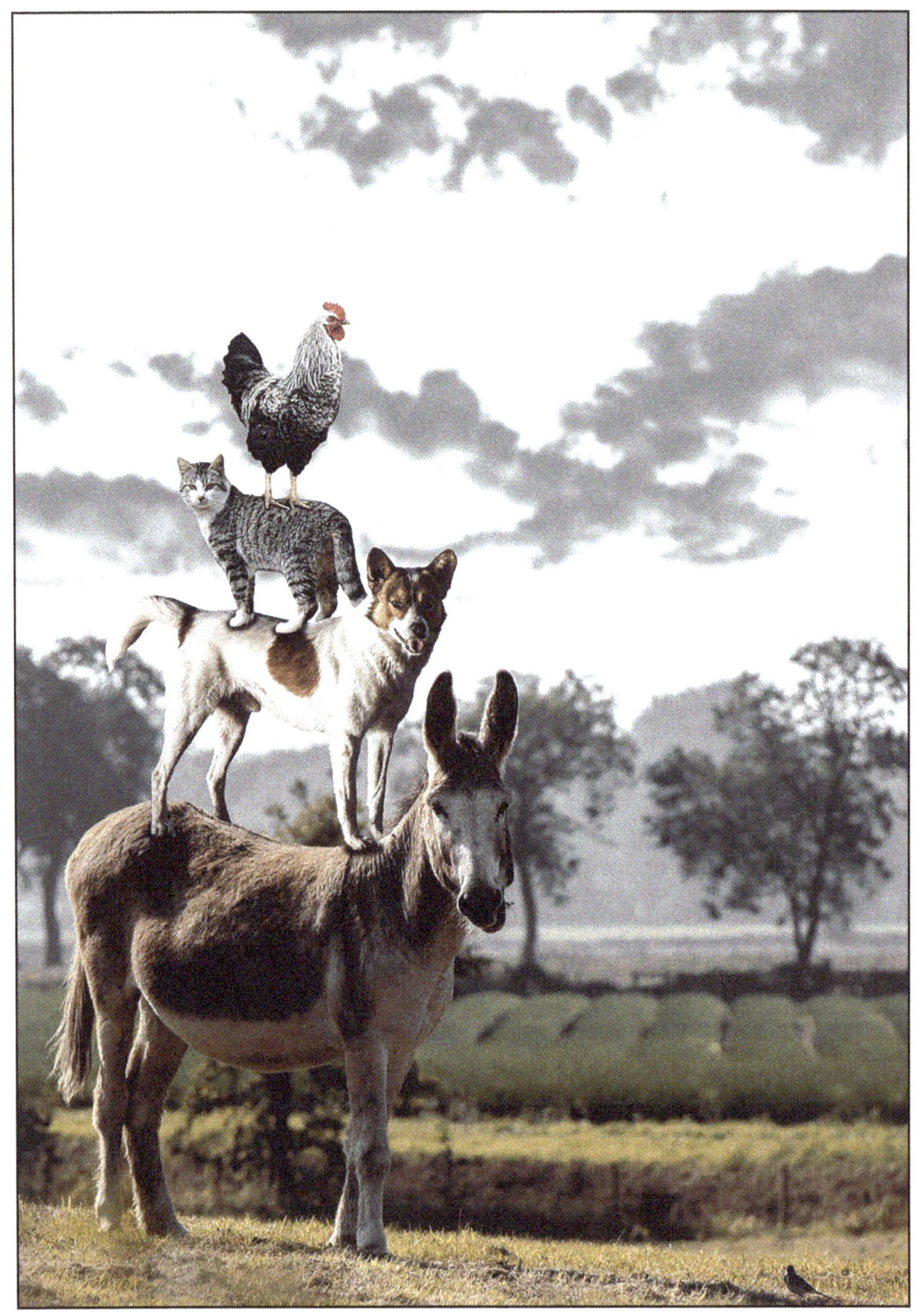

Kirby Was An Animal Scientist

Frances Lebre Smith

There are two years between me and Fran
When she was born I had a second sister
She was named after my paternal Gran
She was so small if you blinked you'd miss her

Her middle moniker came from France
It came from Alsace Lorraine
She could keep you in a trance
Or else drive you insane

I remember her best when she was small
She had hair to her waist and big brown eyes
She surely wasn't afraid of animals at all
And so was closest to Kirby in sibling ties

Yes, she was a real nature lover
She once kept a pet snake
She tried to keep it under cover
Just for propriety's sake

One day while watching TV
Fran patted her overall tog
Ruthie asked, "What's there to see?"
And Fran pulled out a frog

Once Fran took Liebchen for a ride
She took a curve too fast, I want you to know
And the good St Bernard, rather than slide
Did much worse and flew out the window

In addition to her love of creatures
She had an affinity for plants
She knew most plants and their features
Like she knew all her bugs and her ants

She truly has a green thumb
Of this there is no doubt
She'll plant more in days to come
Her advice some folks seek out

When Fran was small she kept a box
In it were all kinds of discarded stuff
If she could have, she'd protect it with locks
She called it her "junks"; castoffs and fluff

I wish I had an inventory list
Of the things she kept in that box
Paperclips, jacks, and a bread bag twist
Were a few of the things, along with some socks

She guarded her "junks" scrupulously
She didn't let just anyone near them
She loaned out items quite judiciously
She rated her "customers", she didn't fear them

One night she took her "junks" to bed
She slept at the time with my older sister
Ruth Helen rolled over on some jacks and said
"Don't bring that stuff to bed or you I'll blister"

The next night Fran wore booties to bed
And about this Ruth Helen asked her
It turns out Fran had it in her head
To stuff the booties with "junks" said Ruth the extractor

Fran was prone to threaten to run away
Whenever there was an altercation
She seldom made it beyond the end of the driveway
She'd return out of sheer desperation

Once she did forsake it
She packed carefully her trunk
Four houses down she did make it
No clothes, no food, only "junks"

Fran was a talented artist
She could sculpt, draw, and paint
In most groups she was the smartest
And is so kind I think she's a saint

Joe Smith

She once painted a dragon for me
It was made completely out of plaster
She painted each scale individually
If I had done it, it would have been a disaster

But when she was done
It was really a true work of art
And, for her, it was fun
Which I knew it would be from the start

She was adept at carving pumpkins
Her jack o' lanterns were simply amazing
They were the envy of the local bumpkins
I kid you not, I can't overdo my praising

She turned her talent into a Fine Arts Degree
She did in four years what took me eight
Attention came naturally, she needn't plea
Her art wasn't just good it was great

She went with the family to Aruba
Were we had an encounter with Dutch Marines
She went us one better by going to Cuba
She was into the international scenes

Time for the wrap up you will agree
We do this you see by degrees
Some of these facts are only a tease
See Fran for details, don't come to me

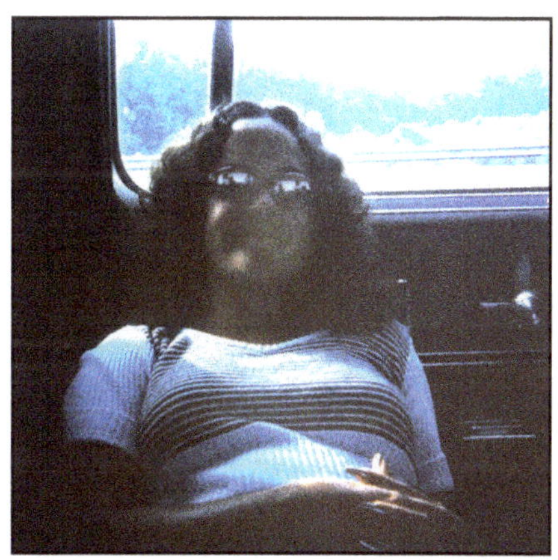

Frances Lebre Smith
on Trip to Aruba - 1975

Frances Was an Artist
Among Other Things

Patricia Marie Smith

This is the tale of my sister Pat
Always industrious from where I sat
When she was a baby she got dehydrated
At the hospital the doctors got frustrated
Finding a vein was found to be impossible
Ankle incisions made infusion possible
This was not the only painful memory
She had a bad burn when she was only three
In an effort to help, she heated up a baby bottle
By putting it on a gas burner and turning it up full throttle
Then without another thought she picked up the nurser
The red hot bottle stuck to her hands, she went no further
She cried out in pain in our mother's arms
Mom did her best to avoid further harm
She bandaged Pat's hands each on its own
Only to find when my father phoned
That each finger should be wrapped separately
To prevent fingers from joining unintentionally
And so unwrapping and re wrapping were required
By this time our mom was getting very tired
From all the effort but mostly from worry
Which had caused her in the first place to hurry
So she unwrapped Pat's hands then wrapped up each finger
She took no time to hesitate or to linger
Meanwhile my sister Ruth, in an attempt to stop the crying
Had fed Pat chocolate bars, Pat's tears to be drying
Unfortunately the result was Pat got ill
On Mom's new couch, I remember that still
Later on Pat went on to obtain a degree in history
What she would eventually do was something of a mystery
She also obtained a psychology degree
Not one to rest, she was busy as a bumble bee
She went on to earn a Masters Degree in Education
Besides that she was certified in School Administration
Just for good measure she minored in math

All these degrees in search of her path
In addition to teacher she was appointed Drug Czar
She obtained a drug sniffing dog to be the star
One day after a fruitless search for drugs
The disappointed dog bit her despite her hugs
Which just goes to show you can't teach a drug dog new tricks
You gotta give 'em drugs if you want to get some licks
In addition to the myriad teaching certifications
She is a certified counselor to increase graduations
Outside of the classroom there was volleyball
And as with her studies she gave it her all
One day while playing she got in the way of a spike
Wound up with double vision, blurriness, and the like
But she wasn't so blind that she couldn't see
A player named Bill Darnell her husband to be
And so you now know of my sister Pat
Who's still Patsy to me despite all of that

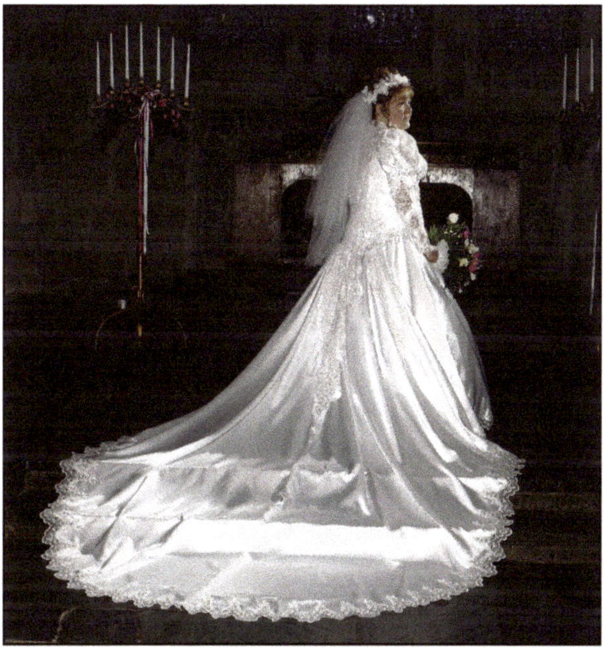

Patsy's Wedding Day
She Was a Teacher

Embroidered Silk
(Benedict Jude)

I have always had four brothers
I thought this was as it should be
I lost one but thankfully no others
I was then left with only three

I only had one brother younger than me
He came to me when I was eight
Thought that was how it always would be
I loved him and thought he was great

I nicknamed him my "Bestus Buddy"
And that's what he always will be
You could say he was my understudy
Not just a blip on our family tree

When he was little I pushed him in a stroller
All the mothers in the neighborhood loved him
I, it seemed, was assigned to be his controller
Happy days as in that stroller I shoved him

When he was only about three years old
He climbed the banister above the first floor landing
And then with a dose of fate so cold
He fell straight down and had a bad crash-landing

My mother held him in her arms
And we prayed he'd be alright
We hoped he'd come to no more harm
As mother held him tight

He was pale and still, almost hypnotized
We thought there could be no worse luck
When suddenly he raised his head and recognized
A familiar sound and called out, correctly, "Truck!"

We knew then that he'd be fine
Was no more worry to it
I never will forget that time
When God saved him I submit

It was about this time, I committed a crime
And took him, crying, from his own bed
I put him in bed with me for a time
As a result he fell, cut his lip, and bled

He had hit the window sill with his chin
And cut completely through his lower lip
Had I obeyed, left him alone, this wouldn't have been
And I would have avoided a lifelong guilt trip

Years later when he lay on his deathbed
I offered a heartfelt apology for this event
"Forgive yourself, for I forgave you long ago" he said
Still to this day my moving him to my bed I lament

When Ben was finally grown
He and my sister came often to visit
Once I owned a home of my own
My children they would babysit

My daughter was crazy about him
That was the main reason I wanted to stay
I was hardly moving away on a whim
But in the end we moved away anyway

We were finally moving away
But the movers hadn't come yet
And so Ben agreed in the house to stay
And I needed to pay with some object

I had an embroidered silk piece of art
It had multi colored flowers Japanese
Ben had said he loved it from the start
Though it was beautiful I gave it with ease

Ben really seemed to like the concept
Of owning this beautiful Japanese piece
And I was glad he was willing to accept
His acceptance gave me some inner peace

Leaving for the West Coast was hard
Leaving Ben alone was even harder
It left my conflicted heart scarred
But I hoped making the move was smarter

Years later when I came to see him
As on his deathbed he lay dying
I prayed that I could guarantee him
I'd get through the visit without crying

My warranty though proved worthless
My emotion just would not be tamed
To my surprise he gave me back mirthless
That Japanese silk which he had had framed

And that was the last I saw of him
On that dreary and fateful day
All alone save the angels above him
As I begged "Dear Lord let him stay!"

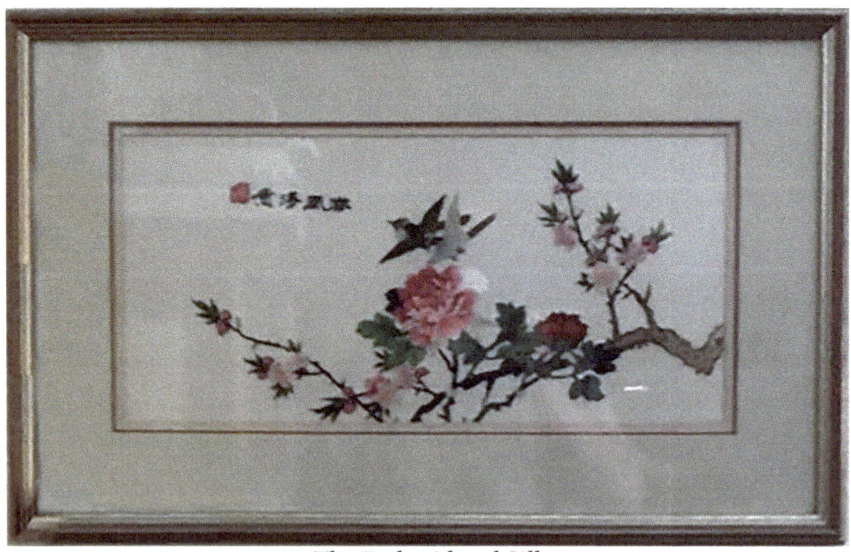

The Embroidered Silk

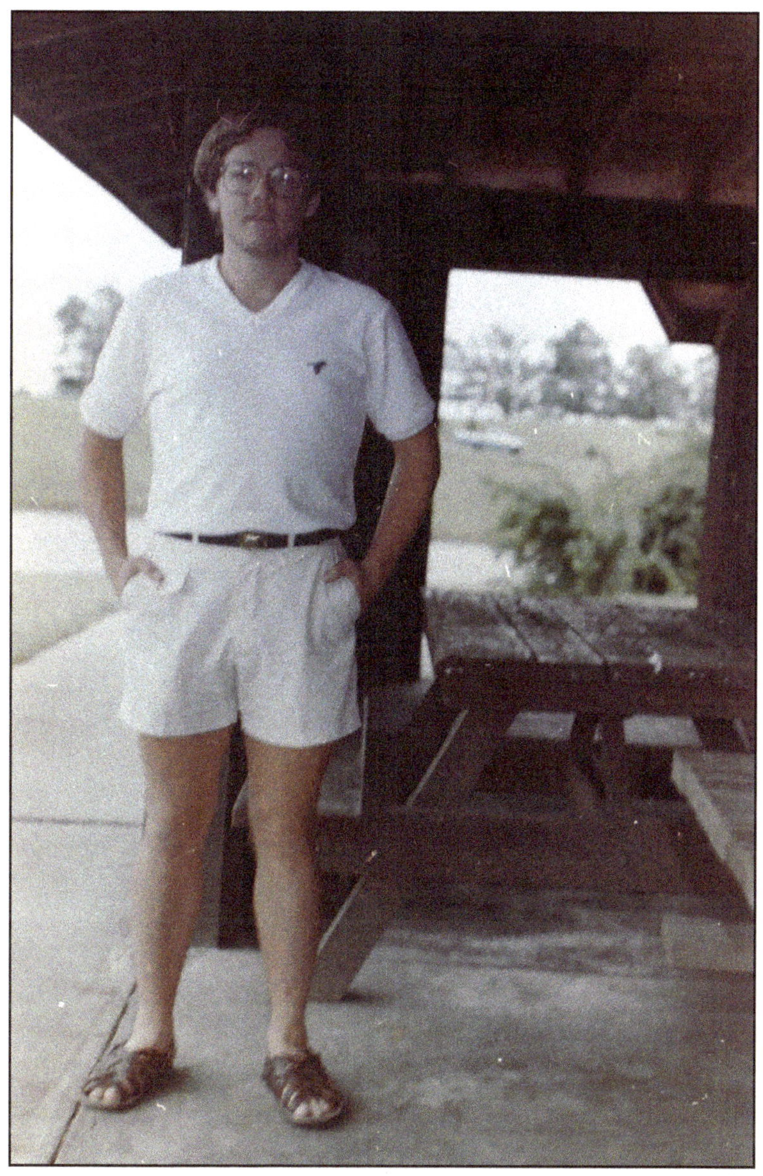

Benedict Jude
He Majored in Business And Worked in The Plastics Industry

Alice's Aliases
(Alice Maureen)

Now is the time to allow for Alice
My sister I claim without malice
She is known as "Number Nine"
Ninth in the line and that is fine
She has had many other appellations
Based on various and sundry situations
She once was called "Alice Blue Gown"
No one who knows why is still around
It appears the name came from the musical "Irene"
But nobody knows if it was derived from "Maureen"
She was named "Alice Maureen" by our Granny
But for awhile she assumed the name "Annie"
"Annie" it seems was a name tied to John Denver
A woman for whom he had feelings tender
When it came time for her to go to school
The school where we all went had a new rule
It seems there would be no first grade
So, for her, other arrangements were made
While eight of us all went to Saint Stephen
Alice alone had to attend public school for a season
So she went to school all on her own
While we were in a group she was all alone
This may have contributed to her independent nature
Which led to her selection as high school drum major
While in high school, Alice learned to play music
Which much later led to careers therapeutic
Given her many monikers it's not surprising
Alice is multi talented in ways of her own devising
She studied and became an X-ray technician
And later added occupational therapy certification
No description of Alice would be complete
Without mentioning dancing, she's light on her feet
She's traveled the region in search of a site
To show off her moves, on her feet as I say, she is light

One other thing I should mention in closing
A characteristic of Alice I am exposing
She's kind to a fault, that I am declaring
She kept my dog for months without swearing
I meant to leave it with her for a short while
Weeks turned into months and still she smiled
I really felt bad about it, in fact I still do
Thus my declaration should be clear to you
And by the way there is one name more
You now call her Al or else she'll get sore
Alice uses nicknames for other relative games
Like Wink and Moe for her sons William and James
And so my story comes to an end
With no more names to append.

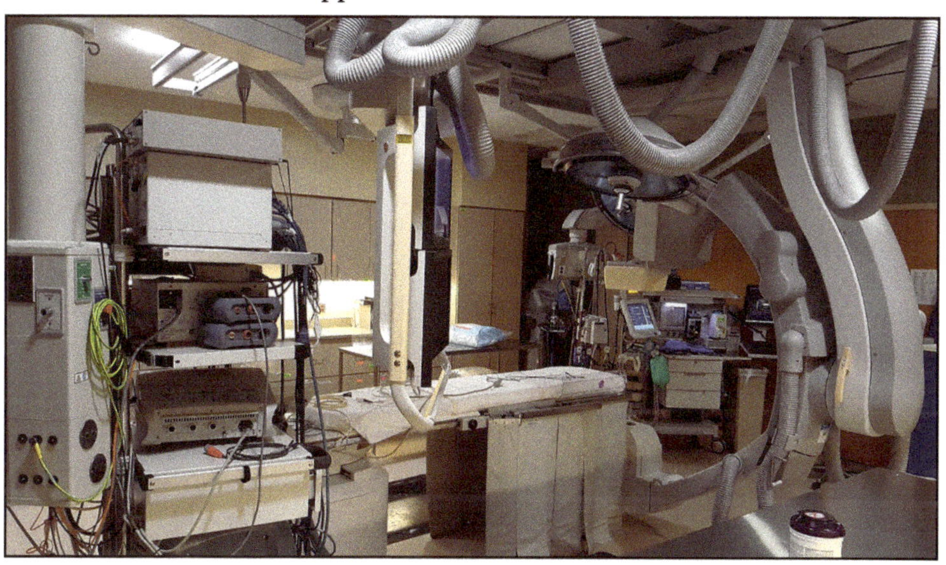

Alice Is An X ray Technician and an Occupational Therapist

A Ferol Tale
(Ferol Teresa)

This is a tale of my sister Ferol
A story of triumph but not peril
You might call it a Ferol Tale
In it I hope to lift the veil

She is a perfect 10
Always has been
10th in birth slot
1st in favored tot

She was a tiny tot, didn't cry a lot
Her affection was sorely sought
Used a stuffed bear for a chair
Learned early on to say a prayer

This is a habit she's long maintained
Served her well as she remained
Faithful to the Golden Rule
Learned before she went to school

In soliciting info for this work
I received notes about her handiwork
All notes mentioned her empathy
Or called to mind her sympathy

She had several nicknames
Not sure who she blames
Dad called her Sugar Foot
He always sought her input

Sparkle Farkle was another name
Before the Farkle name gained fame
On TV's show Saturday Night Live
For originality we did strive

Nurse "Ferd" was another to which she laid claim
She was nursing #8 and #9 when she got this name
On her nurse's hat she spelled out her name
Got the "o" and "l" too close and spelled this new name

Dad didn't tend to show preference
For any child out of deference
To the unique nature of every child
But on Ferol he surely smiled

Ferol proved to be a good student
On academic success she was intent
When it came time for graduation
She came in third in U of L's gradation

She took her degree in Accounting
The anticipation for a CPA was mounting
She took the exam and was successful
She showed she could handle issues stressful

As time went on she gained expertise
She was able to offer guarantees
Full partnership was her next milestone
But to true humility she was still prone

She's the little sister to everybody
And she's a friend to anybody
And most important, all will find
She's the embodiment of kind

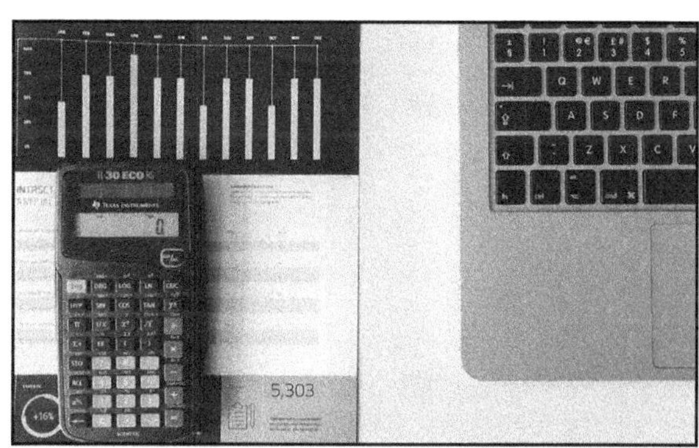

Ferol Is An Accountant

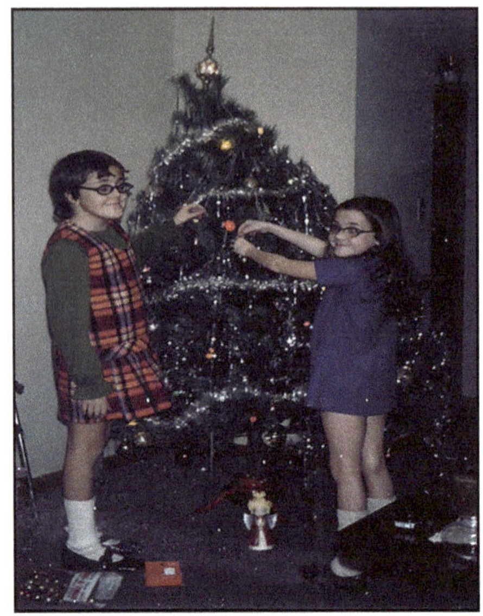

Alice and Ferol Christmas 1970

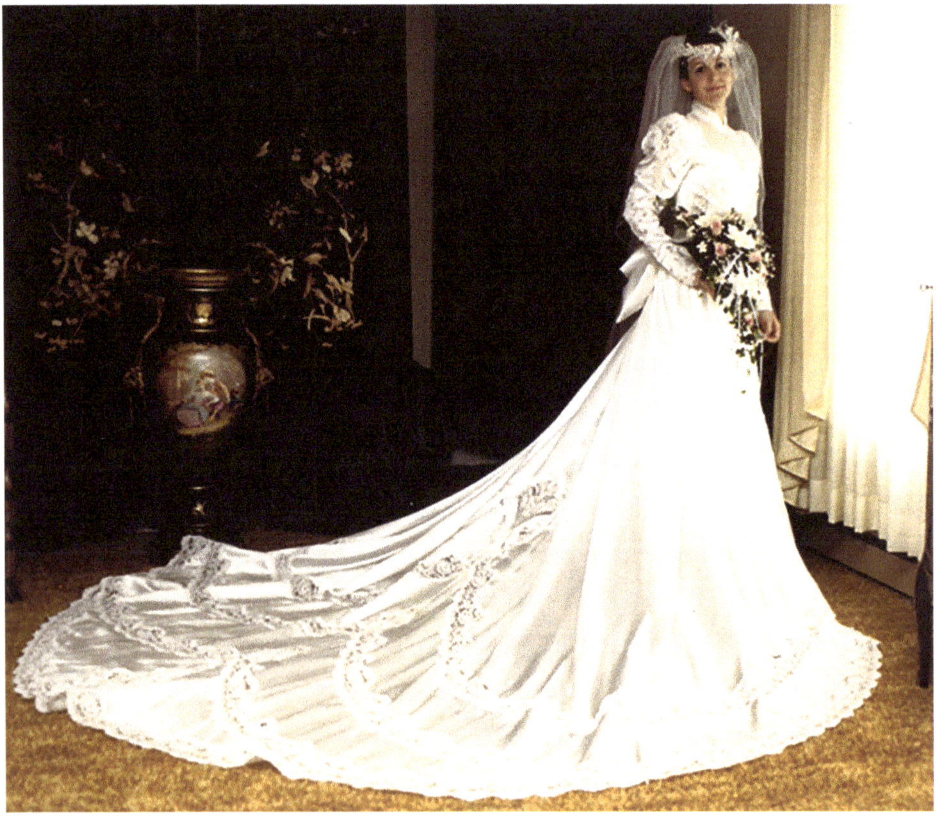

Ferol's Wedding Day

APPENDIX TWO
Simple Observations

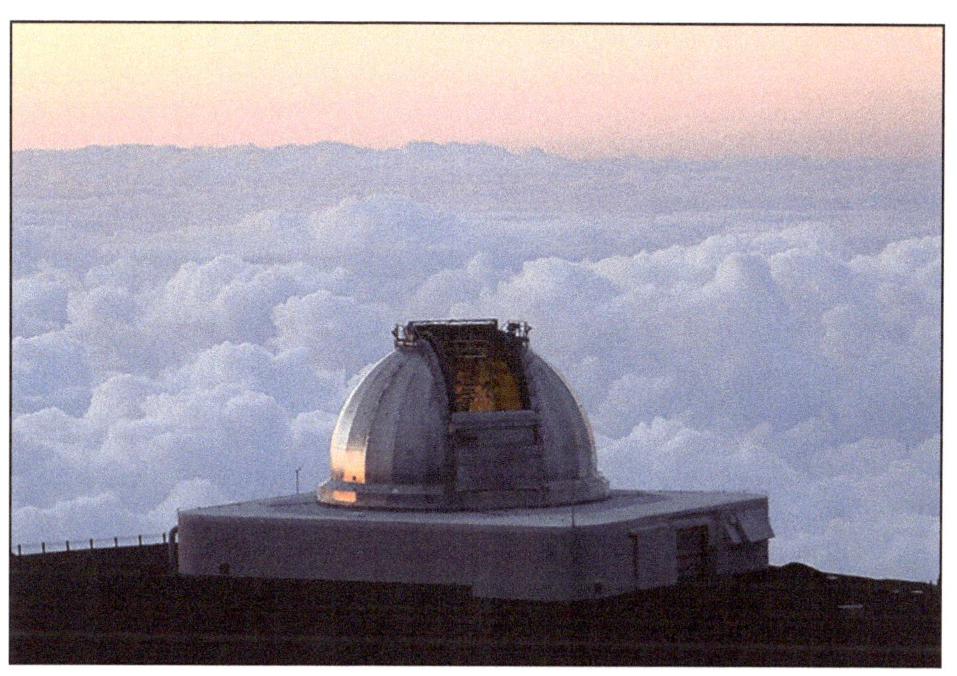

Observatory Observations

Observations

- Repetition Bears Repeating
- Generosity Should Be Given Freely
- Alacrity Should Be Displayed With Enthusiasm
- Felicity Should Be Sought In An Orbit of Happiness
- One Should Avoid Uttering the Word Ineffable
- Ignominious Is A Word To Be Ashamed Of
- One Should Be Protective Of Providence
- Subtlety Cannot Be Emphasized Too Strongly
- Agility Cannot Be Attained Too Clumsily
- Charity, Like Generosity, Should Be Given Freely
- Patience Is Seldom Found Among The Intolerant
- Some people Just Can't Put Up With Longanimity
- Some People Say Redundant Over and Over Again
- When People Want To Show Off They Toss Ostentatious Into The Conversation
- Some People Have The Nerve To Say Audacious
- Perdition Is One Hell Of A Place
- One Should Use The Word Liberality Very Sparingly
- One Should Not Fear The Use Of The Word Valor
- One Should Avoid The Indeterminate Use of The Word Dauntless
- One Should Avoid A Weak Kneed Approach To Fortitude
- Some People Are Ignorant Of The Word Knowledge
- Clarity – I Can't See It
- Some People Think The Word Empyrean Is Just Heavenly
- Sometimes It's Smart To Use The Word Wisdom
- Some Folks Make A Ruckus Over The Word Peace
- Some People Don't Believe In Faith

Helpful Definitions

Alacrity – brisk and cheerful readiness
Felicity – intense happiness
Ineffable – too great or extreme to be described in words
Ignominious – deserving or causing public shame
Providence – the protective care of God or nature as a spiritual force
Subtlety – delicacy
Agility – ability to move quickly and easily
Intolerant – not tolerant of views, beliefs, or behavior that differ from one's own.
Longanimity – patience or tolerance in the face of adversity; forbearance, long suffering
Ostentatious – characterized by vulgar or pretentious display
Audacious – showing an impudent lack of respect
Perdition - (in Christian theology) a state of eternal punishment and damnation into which a sinful and unpenitent person passes after death.
Liberality – the quality of giving or spending freely
Valor – great courage in the face of danger
Dauntless – showing fearlessness and determination
Fortitude – courage in pain or adversity
Empyrean – relating to heaven or the sky

Secondary Observations

- The definitions of cleave are confusing if not downright psychotic
- You can't make short work out of eternity
- Some people can see right through an apparition
- Immensity is no small thing
- A good ascension won't let you down
- Pertinent is a word that doesn't really matter in this case
- The word geriatric is beginning to get old
- Commemorate is a good word to remember
- I'll take equality if it's all the same to you
- I don't care much for apathy
- All this chaos is out of control
- The chapeau has come to a head

- One can only fathom the deep
- You can count your number of fingers on both hands
- You should pay close attention to an annunciation as it can be quite telling
- Anniversaries should be held on an annual basis
- It's not always productive to be on the side of the opposition
- To the beneficiary go the spoils
- An amendment can change everything
- Seniority is old hat
- Remember not to forget
- One should brainstorm the word cerebral
- The word bovine is udderly ridiculous
- Anticipation is worth waiting for
- The Sounds of Silence are deafening
- Contentment is easily endured

Helpful Definitions

Cleave - either to stick together or to split apart
Apparition - a ghost or ghost like image of a person
Immensity - the extremely large size, scale, or extent of something.
Ascension - the act of rising to an important position or a higher level
Pertinent - relevant or applicable to a particular matter
Geriatric - relating to old people, especially with regard to their healthcare.
Commemorate - recall and show respect for (someone or something).
Convention - a way in which something is usually done, especially within a particular area or activity
Apathy - lack of interest, enthusiasm, or concern
Chapeau - a hat
Fathom - n. a unit of length equal to six feet (approximately 1.8 m)
v. understand (a difficult problem or an enigmatic person) after much thought.
Annunciation - the announcement of something
Cerebral - of the cerebrum of the brain
Bovine - relating to or affecting cattle
Contentment - a state of happiness and satisfaction

Joe Smith

Tertiary Observations

- Some of these words are archaic, others are just old and disused
- I made several of these observations while on my matutinal stroll
- The diver refused to go into the water. He was unfathomable.
- Cognitively speaking this is a mindless exercise
- I have heard of people being ambidextrous in both hands
- You just can't make do without the essentials
- The meaning of obscure is somewhat uncertain
- The apprentice asked to be paid in emoluments
- The pain of going through these observations is immitigable
- Although the pain caused by these observations may be immitigable they are assembled sedulously
- The word diurnal came to me during this nocturnal experiment
- We are the posterity of our ancestors
- Statistically speaking probability is a good predictor of outcomes
- H.R. Departments have a difficult job. They have to put together severance packages
- Gangsters tend to be scrupulously unscrupulous
- It's difficult to be premeditated in hindsight
- It's unusual for the obvious to be barely perceptible
- He was resolved to be irresolute
- Small talk is seldom heard in a colloquy
- The poor fellow had an abundance of destitution
- Verdure is a noun that needs to be trimmed back to keep it in its place
- Garfield denies it, but he is a great big grimalkin
- I hold a noncommittal attitude of the pertinacious
- The Sounds of Silence can be obstreperous
- The imp was obsequious to his inner demons
- One seldom looks inward to reach his extremities
- This exercise is meant to be somewhat commoting
- Isn't this just a pretty abomination
- Miniature is a big word for such a small subject

Helpful Definitions

Archaic - very old or old fashioned
Matutinal - of or occurring in the morning.
Unfathomable – incapable of being fully explored or understood; (of water or a natural feature) impossible to measure the extent of.
Cognitively - in a way that relates to or affects cognition.
Cognition - the mental action or process of acquiring knowledge and understanding through thought, experience, and the senses
Essentials - a thing that is absolutely necessary
Obscure - not discovered or known about; uncertain.
Emoluments - a salary, fee, or profit from employment or office.
Immitigable - unable to be made less severe or serious
Sedulously - involving or accomplished with careful perseverance
Diurnal - of or during the day
Posterity - all future generations of people
Scrupulously - in a very careful and thorough way – with great effort to avoid doing wrong
Irresolute - showing or feeling hesitancy, uncertain
Colloquy – a formal conversation
Destitution – poverty so extreme that one lacks the means to provide for oneself
Verdure - lush green vegetation
Grimalkin - a cat (used especially in reference to its characteristically feline qualities)
Pertinacious - holding firmly to an opinion or a course of action
Obstreperous - noisy and difficult to control
Obsequious - obedient or attentive to an excessive or servile degree
Commote - To disturb or agitate, to disrupt also in the positive sense

Joe Smith

Quaternary Observations

- In submitting these lists I am being eleemosynary
- In the interest of modesty, one should repair all holes in one's habiliments
- In using the above two examples I don't mean to be pretentious
- In assuming you'll enjoy this list I may be laboring under a false pretense
- If a ship sails into the Solent Straight, can it be said to be insolent?
- I am certainly ambivalent about the value of these observations
- There is not much substance to the center of an aperture
- I don't know about you, but I think there is something fishy about ichthyology
- There's one thing we can agree on – unanimity
- There is nothing so predictable as the inevitable
- There's nothing that comes so readily as expediency
- Resemblance looks like something, but I can't think what
- Laudable is a word that is praiseworthy
- If I were to call you mendacious, you'd probably call me a liar
- I hope one day to be elected the president of a pantisocracy
- I'd rather be discomposed than decomposed
- There's just no end to the interminable
- It's nearly impossible to blend in conspicuously
- There's nothing quite as certain as a good case of ambiguity
- There is nothing quite as open to company as seclusion
- Dissimilitude is the spice of life
- There's not a legitimate eternity clause in any contract this side of heaven or hell
- Unusual peculiarities are the best kind
- Certain things are inevitable
- Adamantine paradoxically can be broken into syllables*
- There are better things to find yourself in than a predicament

* *Presentation improved by suggestion from Dr Lynn Petras*

Helpful Definitions

Eleemosynary - dependent on charity
Habiliments - clothing
Pretentious - attempting to impress by affecting greater importance, talent, culture, etc., than is actually possessed.
Pretense - an attempt to make something that is not the case appear true.
Solent Straight - a straight in the United Kingdom
Ambivalent - having mixed feelings or contradictory ideas about something or someone.
Insolent - showing a rude and arrogant lack of respect
Aperture - an opening, hole, or gap
Ichthyology - the branch of zoology that deals with fishes
Unanimity - agreement by all involved, consensus
Mendacious - lying
Seclusion - the state of being private and away from other people.
Dissimilitude - dissimilarity or diversity
Pantisocracy - a form of social organization in which all are equal
Discomposed - agitated, disturbed
Dissimilitude - diverse
Adamantine - unbreakable

Joe Smith

Quinary Observations

- It's one thing to find oneself in a quarry, but quite another to find oneself in a quandary
- It is my fervent hope that this list will elicit a cachinnation though some people merely laugh at the word
- If you think about it real hard a cognomen for a person named Nicholas could be seen as redundant.
- You can use the word bodkin to make a point
- My intention in creating these lists is to prevent my becoming mentally torpid
- While I don't want to become torpid, I also want to avoid enervation
- This whole list is supererogatory
- It is sincerely hoped that exposure to this list will not induce the ingestion of ratsbane by the reader
- This list may be seen by some to be an excrescence on the art of literature
- It is inevitable that I should run out of slightly clever ways to use these words
- You can't help but get around circumjacent
- These observations are not great concernments
- There are some who would vituperate me for publishing these observations
- I hope to gain some proselytes to archaic modes of speech by posting these observations
- I hope these observations don't prove to be pernicious, at least not as pernicious as anemia
- Eccentricity is an odd word
- Dolorously is a sad word
- I can't subtilize this exercise anymore than I already have
- I can certainly be accused of casuistry in the propagation of some of these observations.
- While some may accuse me of casuistry I am trying my best to be veracious
- Occur = an Irish hound (Think about it.)

Helpful Definitions

Quandary - a state of perplexity or uncertainty over what to do in a difficult situation.
Cachinnation - a loud or immoderate laugh
Cognomen - an extra personal name given to an ancient Roman citizen, functioning rather like a nickname and typically passed down from father to son.
Duenna - an older woman acting as a governess and companion in charge of girls, especially in a Spanish family; a chaperone.
Bodkin - a small pointed instrument used to pierce cloth or leather.
Torpid - sluggish in functioning or acting
Enervation - a feeling of being drained of energy or vitality; fatigue.
Supererogatory - observed or performed to an extent not enjoined or required; superfluous.
Ratsbane - rat poison, arsenic
Excrescence - a distinct outgrowth on a human or animal body or on a plant, especially one that is the result of disease or abnormality.
Circumjacent - surrounding
Concernments - a matter of interest or importance to someone; a concern.
Vituperate - to blame or insult (someone) in strong or violent language.
Proselytes - a person who has converted from one opinion, religion, or party to another.
Dolorously - causing, marked by, or expressing misery or grief
Subtilize - make more subtle; refine
Casuistry - the use of clever but unsound reasoning
Veracious - speaking or representing the truth.

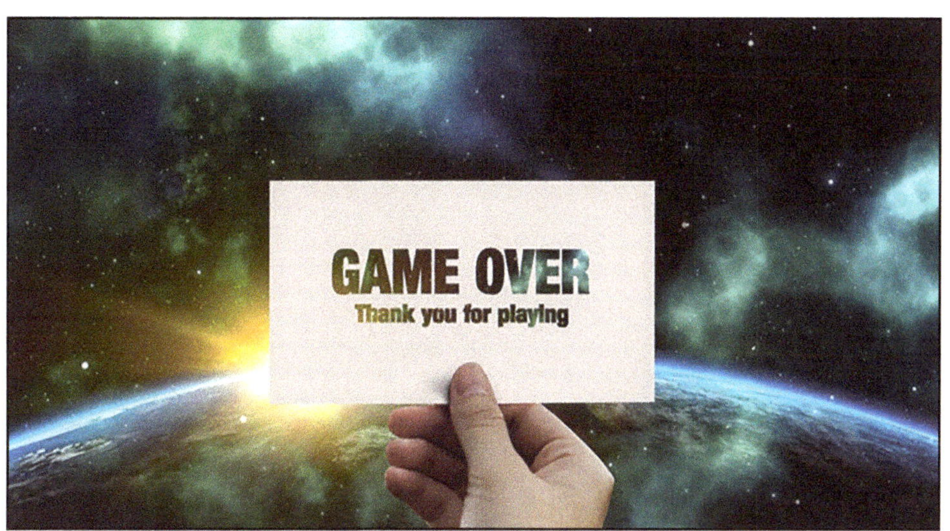

Images are from Pixabay Website or from author's private collection

Minion Pro on 70# LSI Premium Archival White
Type and design by Karen Paul Stone

www.ingramcontent.com/pod-product-compliance
Lightning Source LLC
LaVergne TN
LVHW052345100826
845147LV00012B/754

* 9 7 8 1 9 4 7 5 8 9 7 7 3 *